Happy U:

25 activities to reignite joy
in your yoga practice
and your life

by Olga Kabel, RYT, C–IAYT
Illustrations by Natalia Shkarlet

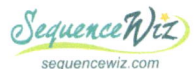

sequencewiz.com

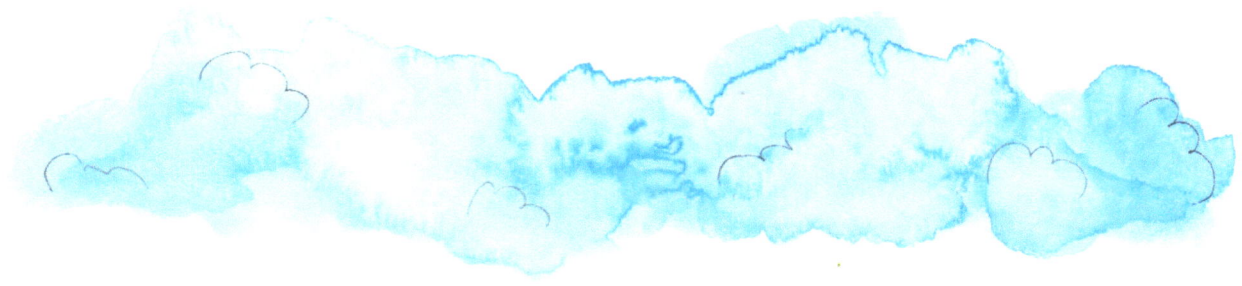

Introduction

Hi there! My name is Olga Kabel. I am a yoga teacher and yoga therapist. I've been practicing and teaching yoga for almost two decades. Over that period of time, my motivation for practicing yoga has changed many times. I have used it to heal my body, manage my energy, inspire my creativity, help me deal with profound life-changing events, and many other reasons. The cool thing about yoga is that it can have a big impact on each area of our lives. Contrary to popular belief, yoga is not just about stretching or strengthening your body; it is actually about directing your energy and clarifying your mind. It also works really well for breaking the inertia of the daily grind and for helping you reassess who you are, where you are in your life, and where you want to be. Another fundamental idea in yoga is that joy is the essence of who we are, but our unruly thoughts, emotions, perceptions, and reactions often obscure this joy. And it is up to us to decide the main emotion we want to live our lives with. Do we want *fear* to rule our lives? Or *anger*? Or *judgment*? Or will it be *joy*? And once we make this decision, we can use our yoga practice to sort through the clutter and unearth our inner joy.

As I get older, I find that it becomes more of an uphill battle to maintain my sunny disposition because with life experience comes an accumulation of scars from the past, stories of other people's suffering, and fears about the wellbeing of my own family and community. Most of the time, these fears never materialize, but they can still ruin a perfectly good day (or several). One quote I keep coming back to goes, "Worrying does not take away tomorrow's troubles. It takes away today's peace." It takes consistent effort to keep worry at bay, and I find that yoga helps with this the most.

From an evolutionary standpoint, our brains are wired to be suspicious and expect the worse. This served us well in terms of the survival of the species, but it doesn't work so well if you are trying to minimize the amount of stress and worry in your life. Luckily, within our same brains, we have neurocircuitry dedicated to the feelings of peace, contentment, and joy. This reminds me of a story from the Elizabeth Berg's novel, *The Year of Pleasures*. In it, a Navajo grandfather tells his grandson this story: "'Two wolves live inside me. One is the bad wolf, full of greed and laziness, full of anger and jealousy and regret. The other is the good wolf, full of joy and compassion and willingness and a great love for the world. All the time, these wolves are fighting inside me.' 'But grandfather,' the boy asked. 'Which wolf will win?' The grandfather answered, 'The one I choose to feed.'"

In this journal, I've compiled 25 simple activities you can do to "feed the joyful wolf." They include simple tasks, reflections, and occasional yoga practices to counterbalance the brain's negative bias and make a more positive outlook the new normal. Some activities are only few minutes long; others will involve simply looking at your hurdles in a new light, and others will be full-length yoga practices—you get to pick what fits into your life right now. These small steps have the potential to shift how your brain responds to obstacles and rewire it to experience the world from a calmer and happier place.

Each activity presented in this journal includes the reason for doing it as well as specific instructions on how to integrate it into your life. Some of those activities are derived from books that inspire me (you can find the full list in the References section), and others were compiled from my own experience as well as from feedback from my yoga students. I suggest that you do each activity at least once a day for a week to see if it makes a difference in how you engage with your life. Many activities include additional free content that you can find at happyuhub.com/journal. The website includes videos of yoga practices, blog posts on related topics, informational handouts, and other fun materials. Please check out this content to enhance your experience.

By themselves, yoga practices don't mean anything; they only become meaningful when you use them as tools to achieve whatever you want to achieve. One of my students once said to me, "I just want to be healthy and happy." Isn't this what we all want? So let's try to figure out how we can use yoga and awareness to make ourselves healthier and happier on a daily basis. We will do this by figuring out what it means to you to be happy, and we will take small, specific steps to enhance your life and brighten your outlook.

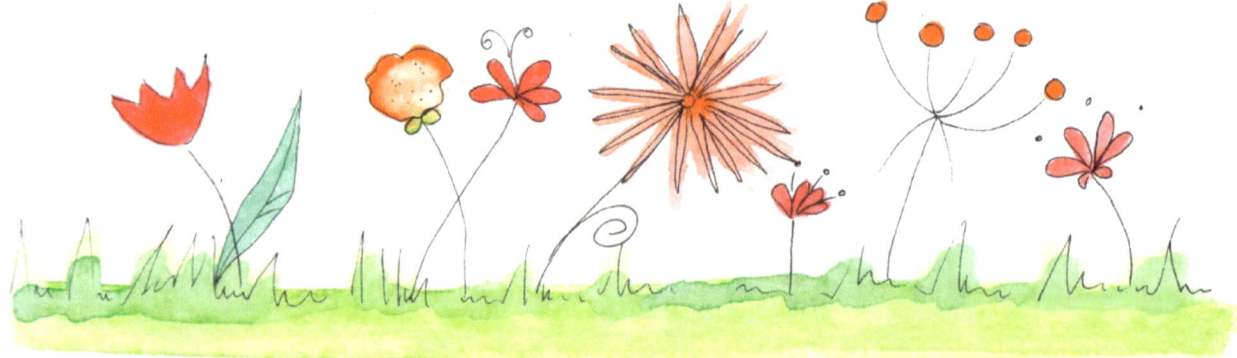

Happiness is
a direction,
not a place

Check in: are you breathing?

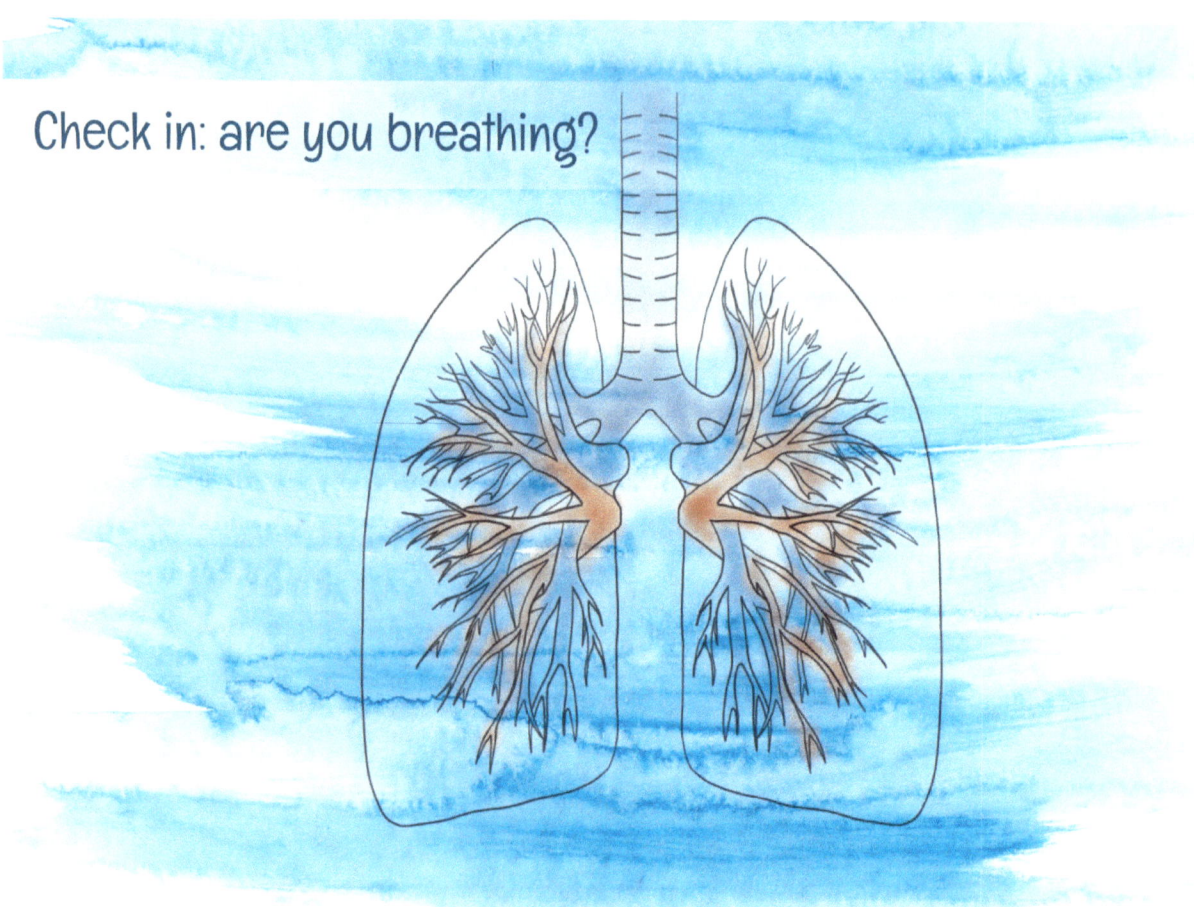

The quality of your breathing accurately reflects the state of your sympathetic nervous system (SNS): fight-or-flight response leads to short, fast breaths bordering on hyperventilation, while rest-and-digest activation leads to deep relaxed breathing. And it works the other way around, too: short, shallow breath is perceived by the brain as an invitation to fight or flee, while slow, deep breathing is viewed as an invitation to rest and digest.

HOW TO: Take a few moments throughout your day to notice the quality of your breath and what it says about the state of your sympathetic nervous system. If you find yourself holding your breath or taking short, restrictive breaths at any point, relax your body, take three full deep breaths, and notice how it makes you feel.

🖱 Additional content: Why bother with breath? (pdf handout)

NOTES

"If you can breathe, you can do yoga."
— Sri Krishnamacharya

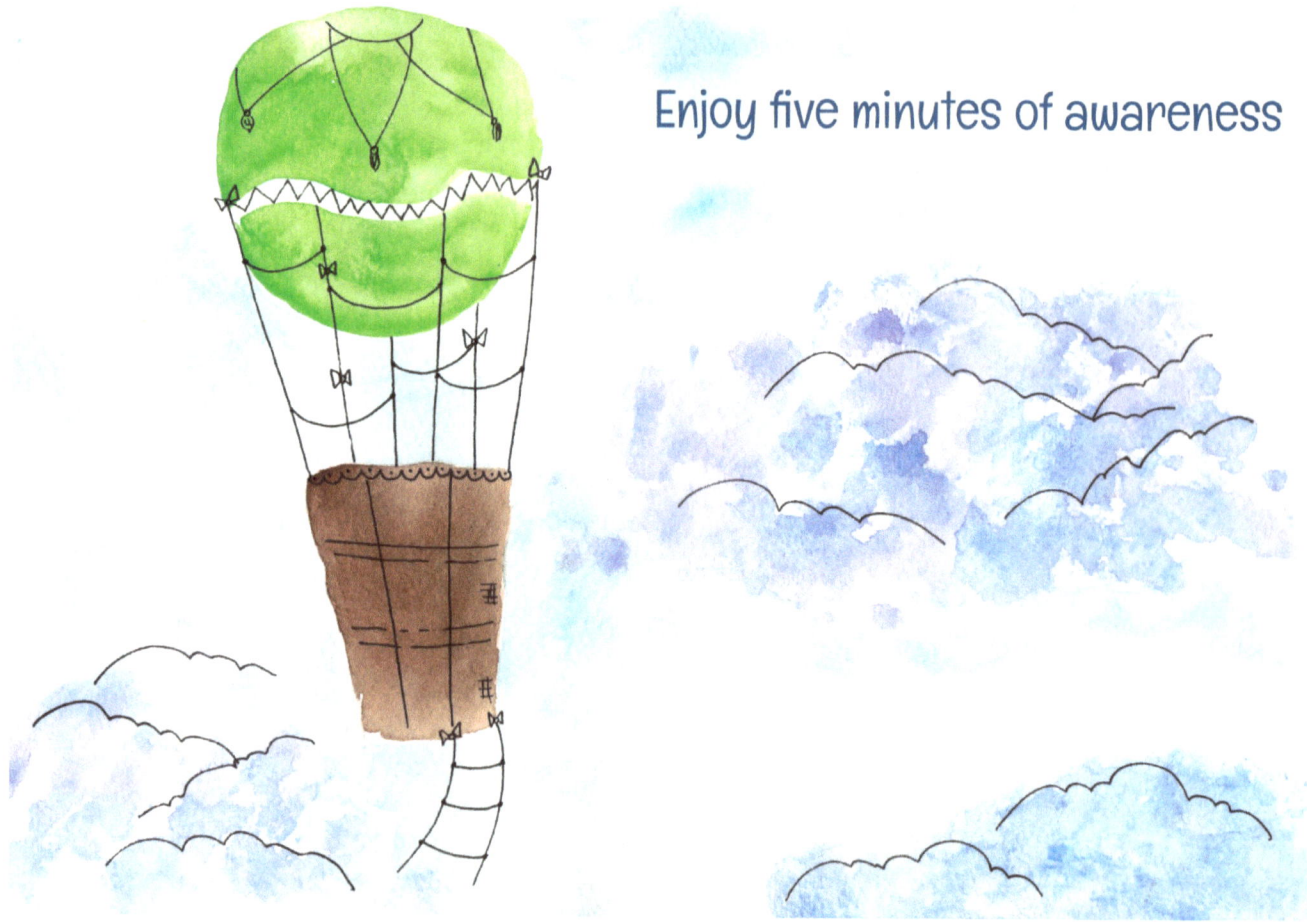

Enjoy five minutes of awareness

During the day, we are mostly externally oriented: we pay attention and respond to things that are happening around us. We perceive the world through our senses – it's called *perception*. But it is just as important to cultivate *interoseption* — an ability to perceive and interpret our physiological sensations — to gain a better understanding of the impact that the external world has on our mood, physiology, and health.

HOW TO: Get settled in a comfortable seated position and close your eyes. Notice how your body feels and the flow of your breath. Take a mental note of the state of your mind. How are you doing in this particular moment? Do you feel rushed, centered, or lethargic? Don't do anything about it; just pay attention to it for five minutes. How do you feel afterwards?

🖱 Additional content: Short uplifting yoga practice (video)

NOTES

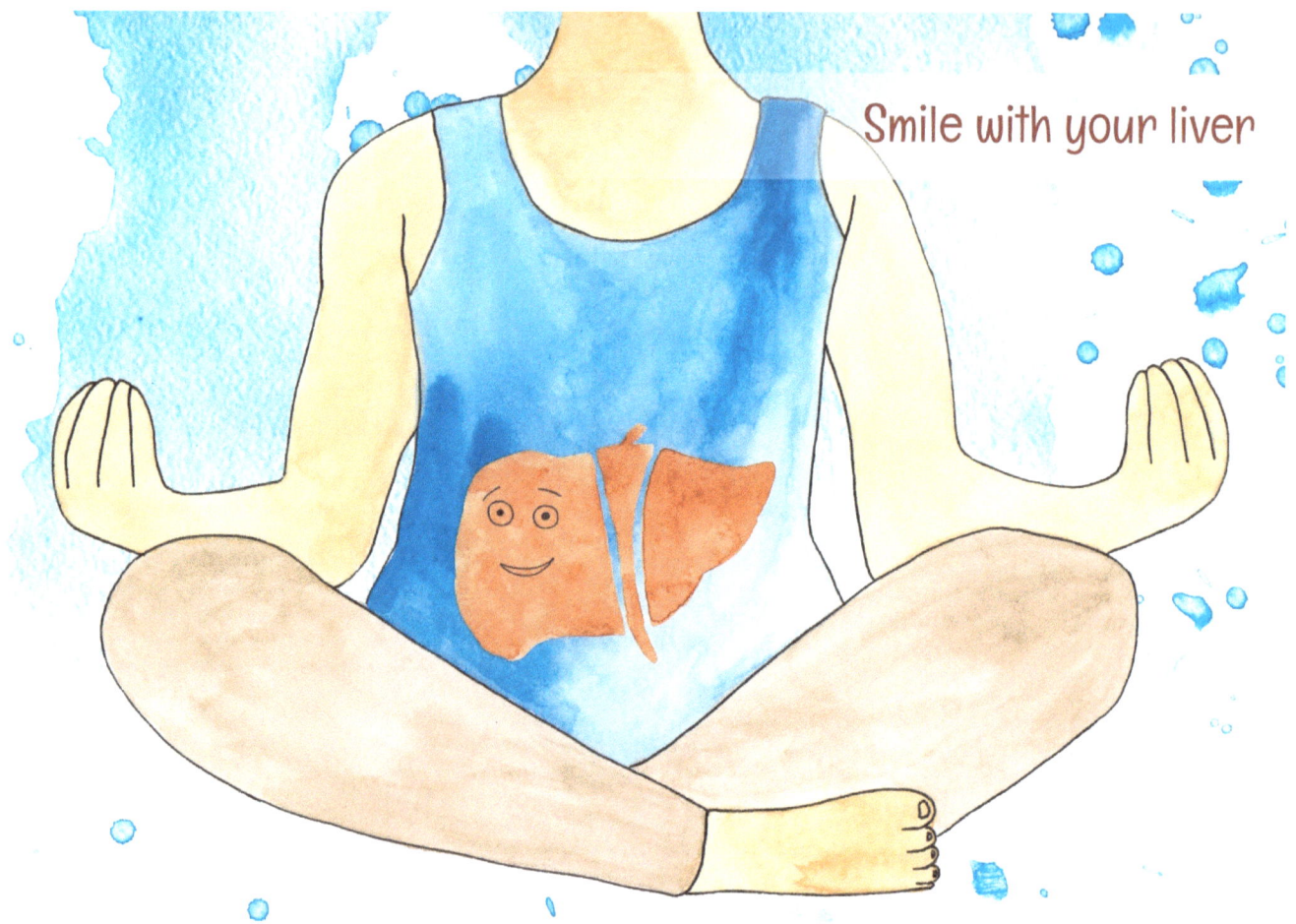

Smile with your liver

In Elizabeth's Gilbert's memoir *Eat, Pray, Love*, her spiritual teacher in Bali encourages her to lighten up a bit by smiling with her liver while meditating. He says: "Why they always look so serious in Yoga? You make serious face like this, you scare away good energy. To meditate, only you must smile. Smile with face, smile with mind, and good energy will come to you and clean away dirty energy. Even smile in your liver."

HOW TO: Get settled in a comfortable seated position and close your eyes. Notice how your body feels, the flow of your breath, and then take a mental note of the state of your mind. Then bring your attention to the right side of your body toward the bottom of the ribcage. This is where your liver is. Take few breaths focusing on that area and then imagine your liver smiling. Continue to smile with your liver for five minutes.

🖱 Additional content: Short uplifting yoga practice (video)

NOTES

Laugh every day

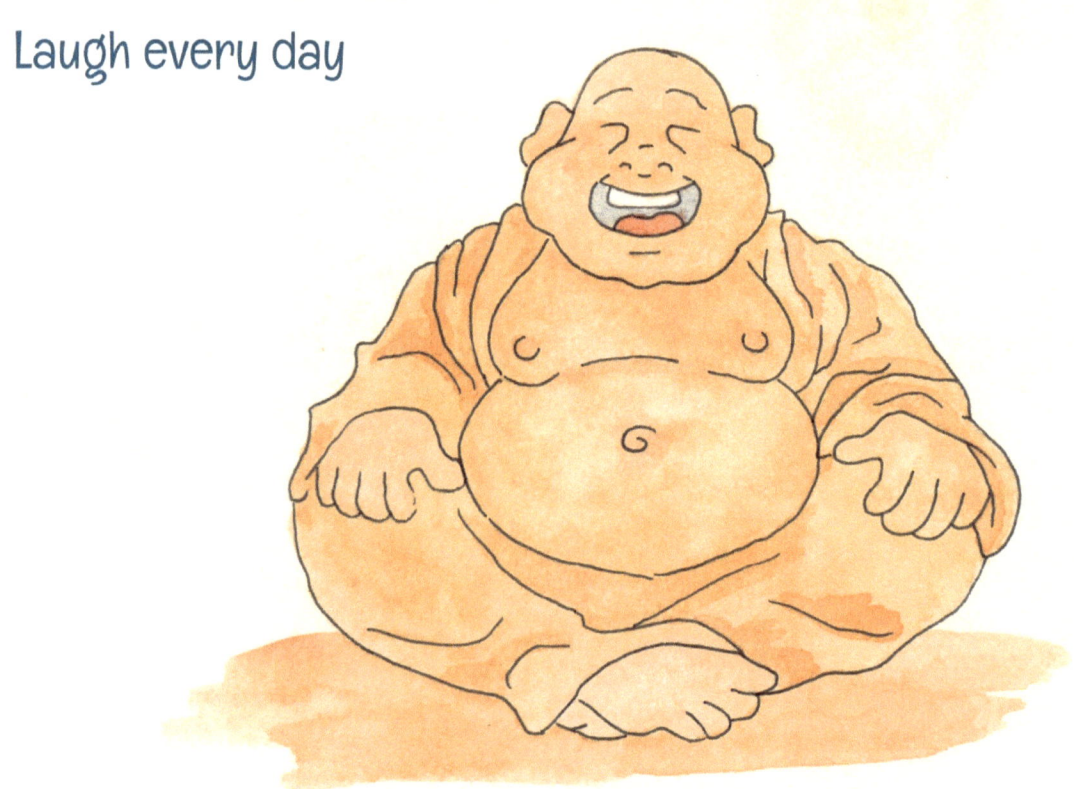

We all know that the goal of yoga is to quiet the mind. What happens to your mind when you laugh? It becomes silent. According to some yogis, this is true yoga. Steve Ross in his book *Happy Yoga* asks: "Do you ever laugh so hard you get dizzy and tingly? If you don't, you are not having enough fun. [...] From just a little giggle, your body is flooded with biochemicals, including neurotransmitters and endorphins, that can elevate mood, alleviate depression, and relieve stress."

HOW TO: Figure out what kind of things make you laugh. Do you like cartoons? Comedy shows? Funny books? Funny friends? Be sure to get your dose of laughter from those sources every day and don't hold back on your reactions — laugh like you mean it!

Additional content: Yoga fun (collection of cartoons)

NOTES

"It is a curious fact that people are never so trivial as when they take themselves seriously."
— Oscar Wilde

Practice the Superwoman stance

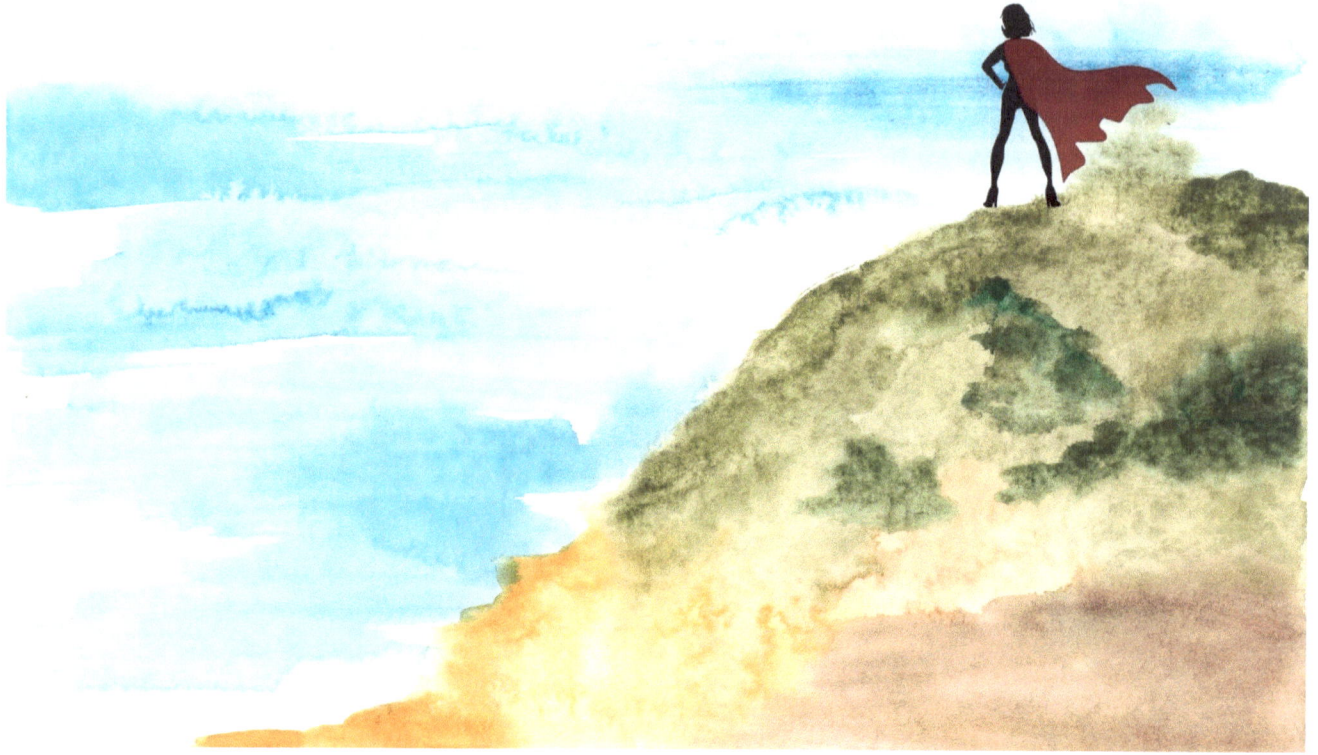

The way we carry our bodies in our daily lives affects the way we feel. Open, expansive postures, similar to the Superwoman stance, make us feel assertive, powerful, and confident; they decrease anxiety and make us more optimistic. Amy Cuddy, the author of the book *Presence* writes: "Your physical posture sculpts your psychological posture, and could be the key to a happier mood and greater self-confidence."

HOW TO: Stand tall with your feet slightly wider than hip distance apart. Place your hands on your hips, relax the shoulders, and look directly in front of you. Breathe deeply. With every inhalation, imagine yourself growing a little taller, and with every exhalation, imagine yourself becoming a bit more grounded. Hold your head up high and stay aware of your surroundings without focusing on anything specific. Take 12 breaths like that.

⌒🖱 Additional content: Superwoman warm-up (video)

NOTES

Spend time outside

Some years ago, I read an interview with Oprah, in which she mentioned one of the main reasons she decided to wrap up her Chicago show and move to California. She said that for years, she barely spent any time outside! Every morning she would step from her house into the car, to the parking garage of her studio, and then to her studio; in the evening, she did the same in reverse. We are not Oprah, but we can easily get into the same rhythm and barely go outdoors. This can have a profound narrowing impact on our outlook.

HOW TO: Spend at least 30 minutes outside every day moving. It doesn't have to be all at once, and it doesn't matter what you do — walk, tend to your garden, shovel snow — just move your body. When you go outside, notice the feeling in your body, the quality of your energy, as well as the state of your mind. Gradually, work on organically building it into your day.

NOTES

Give thanks: three gratitudes

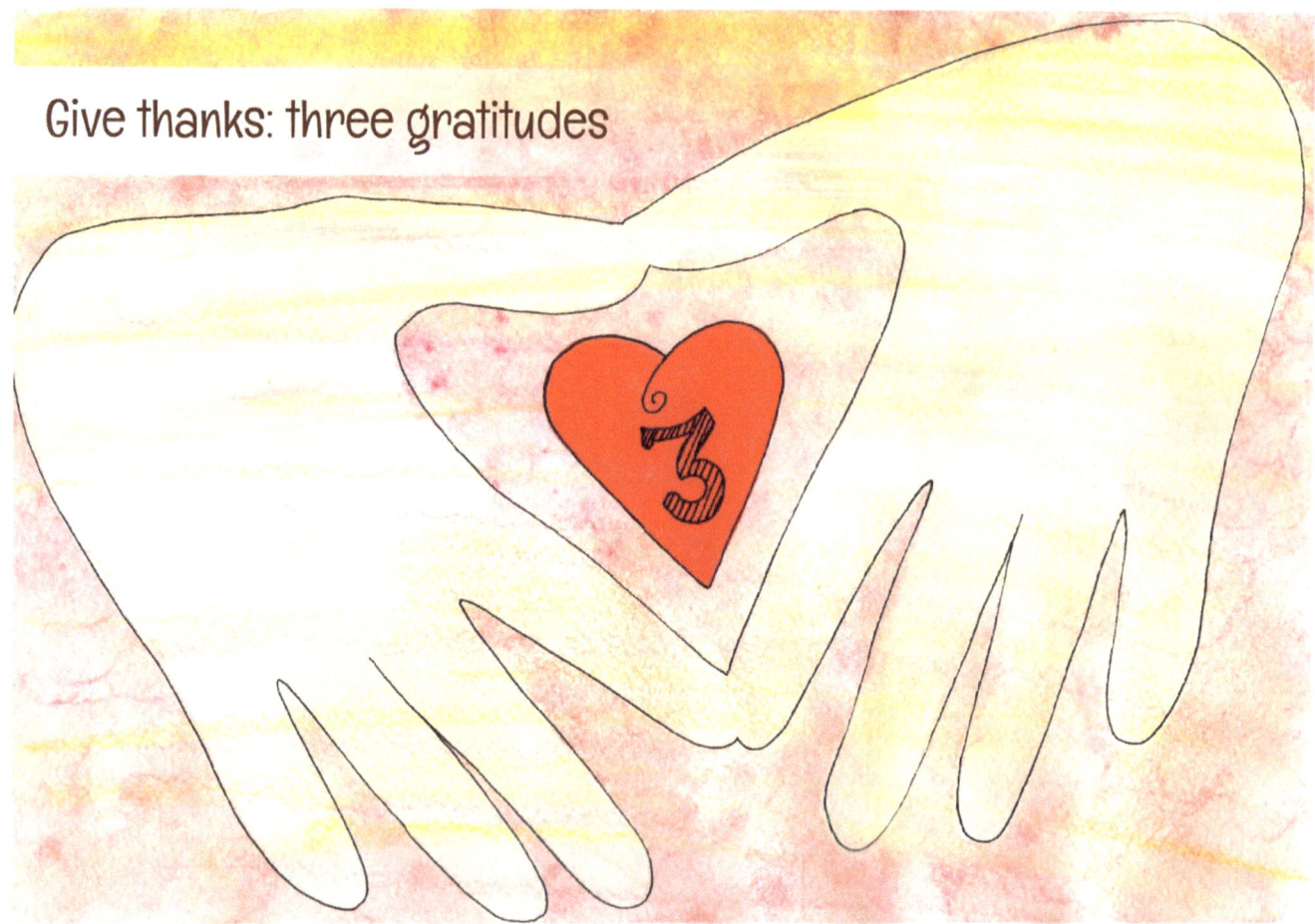

In his book *The Happiness Advantage*, Shawn Achor describes how expressing gratitude for three specific things every day shifts the way your brain perceives the world. Normally, your brain scans the world for potential dangers. But if you get in a habit of noticing just three good things that happened, your brain develops a pattern of scanning the world for the positive instead. When you notice the positive and acknowledge it by expressing gratitude, you begin to perceive your circumstances in a very different way.

HOW TO: Every day write down three specific good things that just happened and express gratitude for them. Make those things different every day. You can make it a solitary activity, or you can include other members of your family by asking them to share three things they are grateful for at dinner time, for example.

🖱 Additional content: Gratitude yoga practice (video)

NOTES

"The Mind is its own place, and in itself can make a heaven of hell, a hell of heaven."
— John Milton

Master your Zorro circle

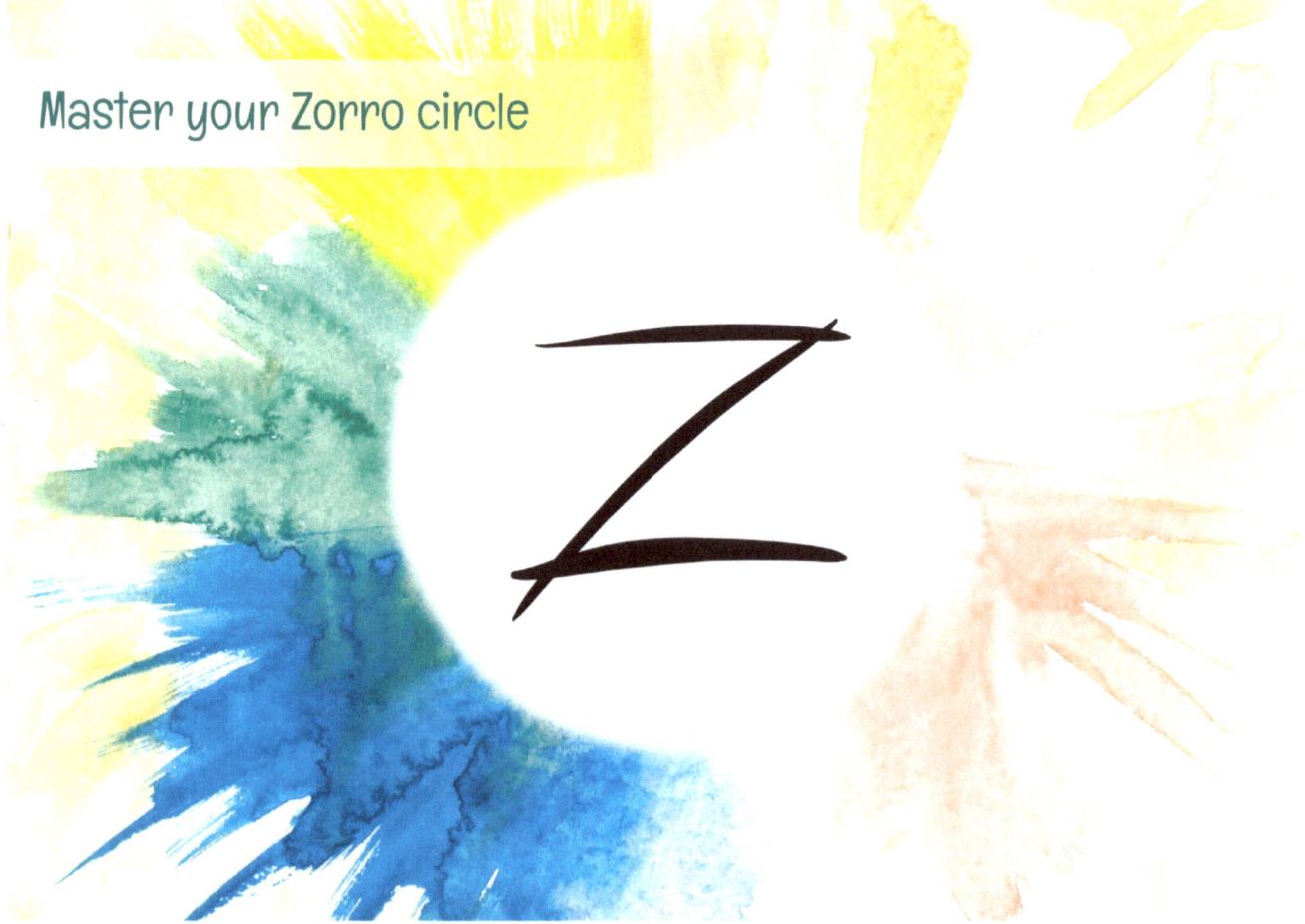

In the legend of Zorro (as described by Shawn Achor in *The Happiness Advantage*), young, passionate, and undisciplined Alejandro wants to fight villains and right the injustices in the world, yet he wants to do it all at once and fails spectacularly. After many heroic attempts and many failures, he feels utterly disillusioned and powerless. This is when the aging sword master Don Diego finds him and recognizes his potential. To begin Alejandro's training, Don Diego draws a circle in the dirt and allows him to fight only within that circle. Only after Alejandro masters control of this circle is he allowed to undertake bigger and bigger challenges. Before long, he is swinging on chandeliers and winning all sorts of sword fights. But this would never have been possible if he hadn't learned how to master that small original circle. The moral of the story is that to achieve anything in life, we need to focus our efforts on small manageable goals, which, once accomplished, give us a sense of control and fuel our desire to continue.

HOW TO: Identify an area of your life where you are struggling or feel overwhelmed. Is it some aspect of your work? Your relationships? Your health? Draw a small circle and write the problem in the middle of it. Then draw a bigger circle around it — this is your circle of control (the Zorro circle). What do you have control over in this situation? Write those things down within the circle. What don't you have control over? Write those things down outside of the circle. Then look at it and reflect on how you can improve the things that are in your control. How can you master your Zorro circle? What steps can you take?

Additional content: sample Zorro circle

Change a habit

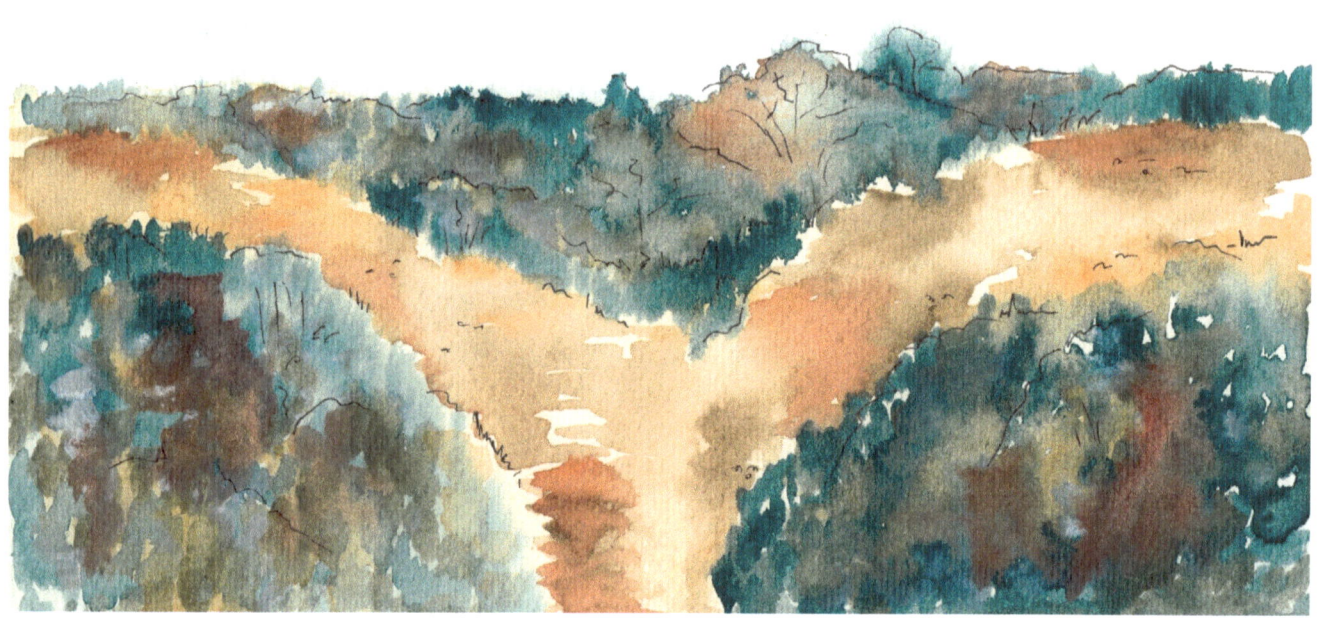

You probably have some habits that you would like to change, yet you know how difficult it is. A key to breaking an old habit and replacing it with a new one is intentionally making it as easy as possible to do the new thing and as hard as possible to do the old thing. Want to read more books and watch less TV? Hide your remote and put a book in its place on your coffee table. Want to eat healthier? Replace all unhealthy items with healthy ones in your fridge. Which habit do you want to break?

HOW TO: Identify a habit that is not serving you well. It can be a habit in any area of your life (health, wellness, work, relationships, fun, etc.). What would you like to replace it with? What concrete steps can you take to make the old behavior harder and the new behavior easier to do? Take those steps to set yourself up for success and engage in the new behavior for a week.

🖰 Additional content: How to build a habit of consistent and meaningful home yoga practice (blog post)

NOTES

"Information is not transformation."
— Shawn Achor *The Happiness Advantage*

Notice your itty bitty s#*&&y committee

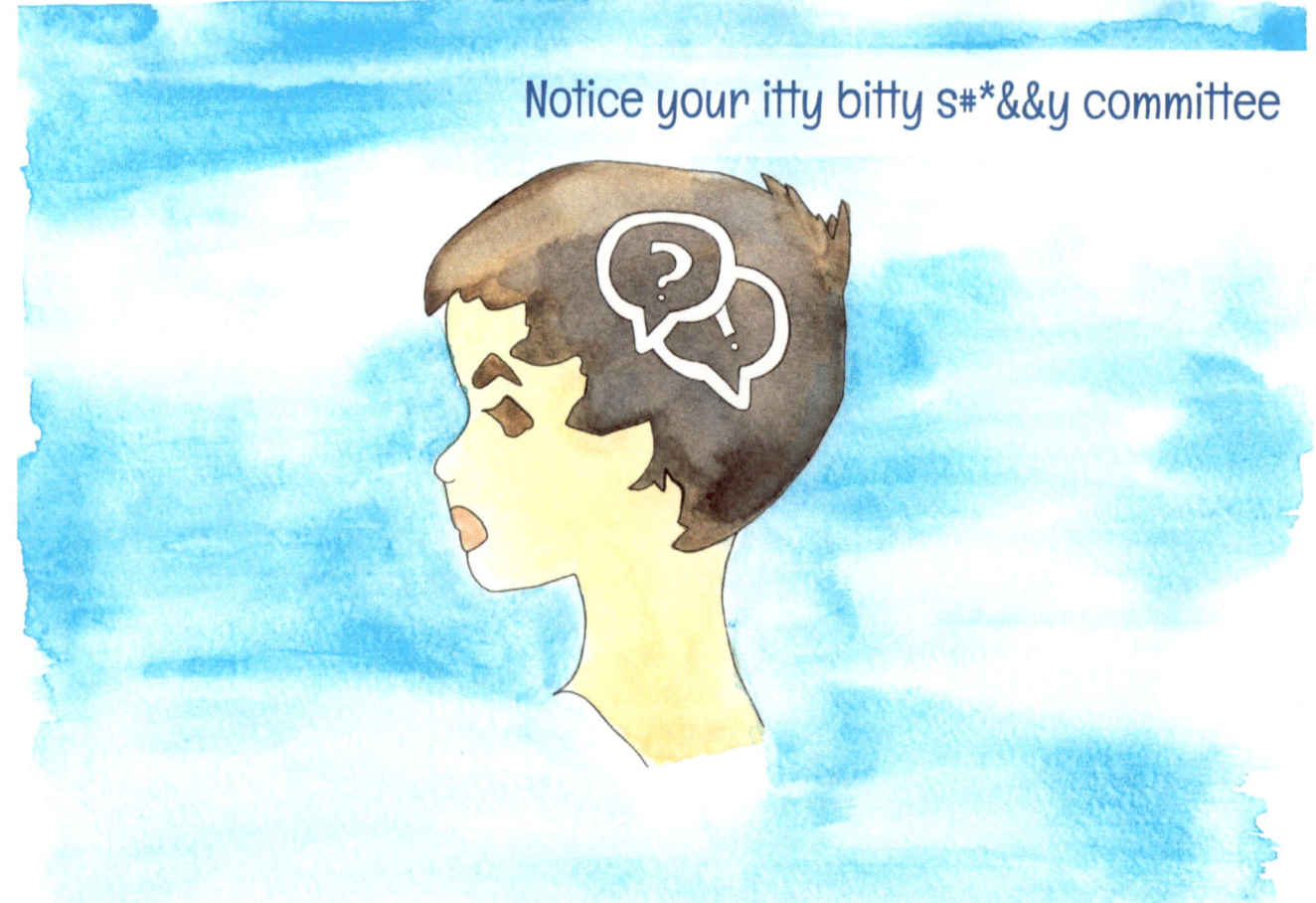

The vast majority of cells in your body work tirelessly around the clock to keep you healthy, happy, and successful. But there is a small group of cells in our brains that seems to be committed to sabotaging our best efforts and sense of inner joy. As Jill Bolte Taylor says in her book *My Stroke of Insight,* "these cells tap into our negative attributes of jealousy, fear, and rage. They thrive when they are whining, complaining, and sharing with everyone how awful everything is." This group of cells has been called many names, including "The Itty Bitty S#*&&y Committee."

HOW TO: Notice the complaining voice in your mind that likes to air out big and small grievances both in your daily life and during your yoga practice. Don't do anything about it, just take note: "Here you are again. What are you dissatisfied with now?" Notice if you have recurring loops of grievances that keep coming up again and again, and notice how thinking like that makes you feel.

NOTES

Hum for mental clarity (bee breath)

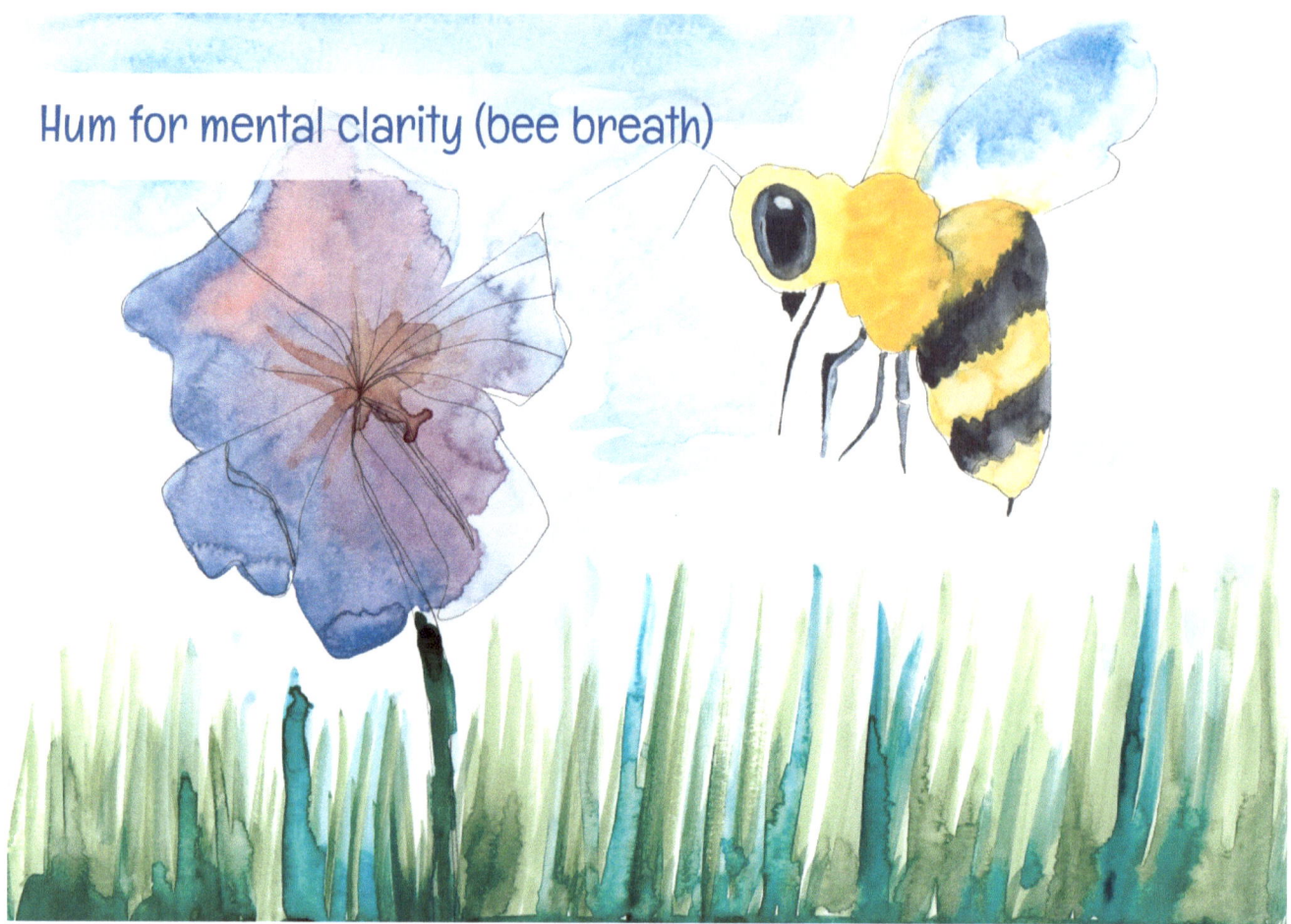

Studies show that chanting OM promotes limbic deactivation, which means that it takes the edge off our basic emotions (fear, pleasure, and anger) and drives (hunger, sex, dominance, and care of children). This confirms a yogic idea that chanting has a discharging effect on the brain, meaning that it discharges us from compulsive thinking, wanting, and grasping, which may be happening because of the stimulation of the vagus nerve during vocalization. Bhramari Pranayama (bee breath) has a similar effect.

HOW TO: Take a deep breath and then exhale slowly as you make a long low-pitch one-tone M sound. Continue to breathe like that and focus on the vibration in your throat and around the ears as you hum. Repeat for 12 breaths.

🖰 Additional content: bee humming breath (video) + blog post about humming and chanting

NOTES

Practice the 90-second rule

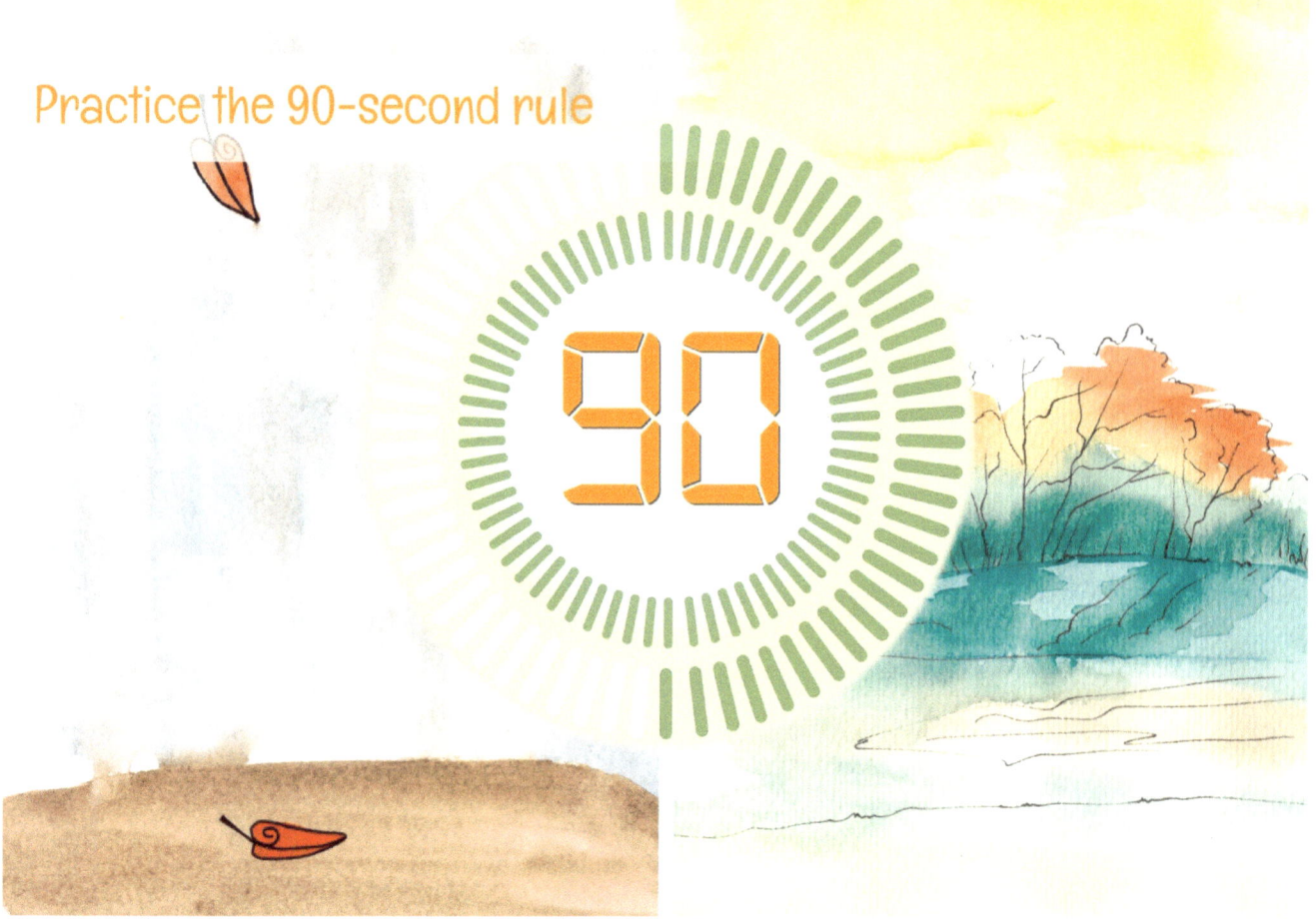

In her book *My Stroke of Insight*, neuroscientist Jill Bolte Taylor states that it takes about 90 seconds for a strong emotional response to travel through your entire system: "Although there are certain limbic system (emotional) programs that can be triggered automatically, it takes less than 90 seconds for one of these programs to be triggered, surge through our body, and then be completely flushed out of our blood stream." This means that any programmed response — anger, for example —gets triggered automatically and produces a surge of chemicals that makes up a physiological experience. But within 90 seconds, that physiological experience has come and gone. Dr. Bolte Taylor continues: "If, however, I remain angry after those 90 seconds have passed, then it is because I have CHOSEN to let that circuit continue to run. Moment by moment, I make the choice to either hook into my neurocircuitry or move back into the present moment, allowing that reaction to melt away as fleeting physiology."

HOW TO: Next time when you have a strong emotional reaction to something, give it 90 seconds to wash over you. Don't fight it, just notice. After about 90 seconds, remind yourself that you have a choice now to either hold on to that emotion or to pull yourself out of it. And then make that choice. You can continue to stew in the emotion, if that's your choice, or you can anchor your attention in the present moment by focusing on one of your senses (sight, smell, tactile sensations, etc.) or breathing. Notice if you succeed in breaking the emotional loop.

NOTES

"Finding the balance between observing our circuitry and engaging with our circuitry is essential for our healing."
Jill Bolte Taylor, *My Stroke of Insight*

Rub your tummy, pat your head

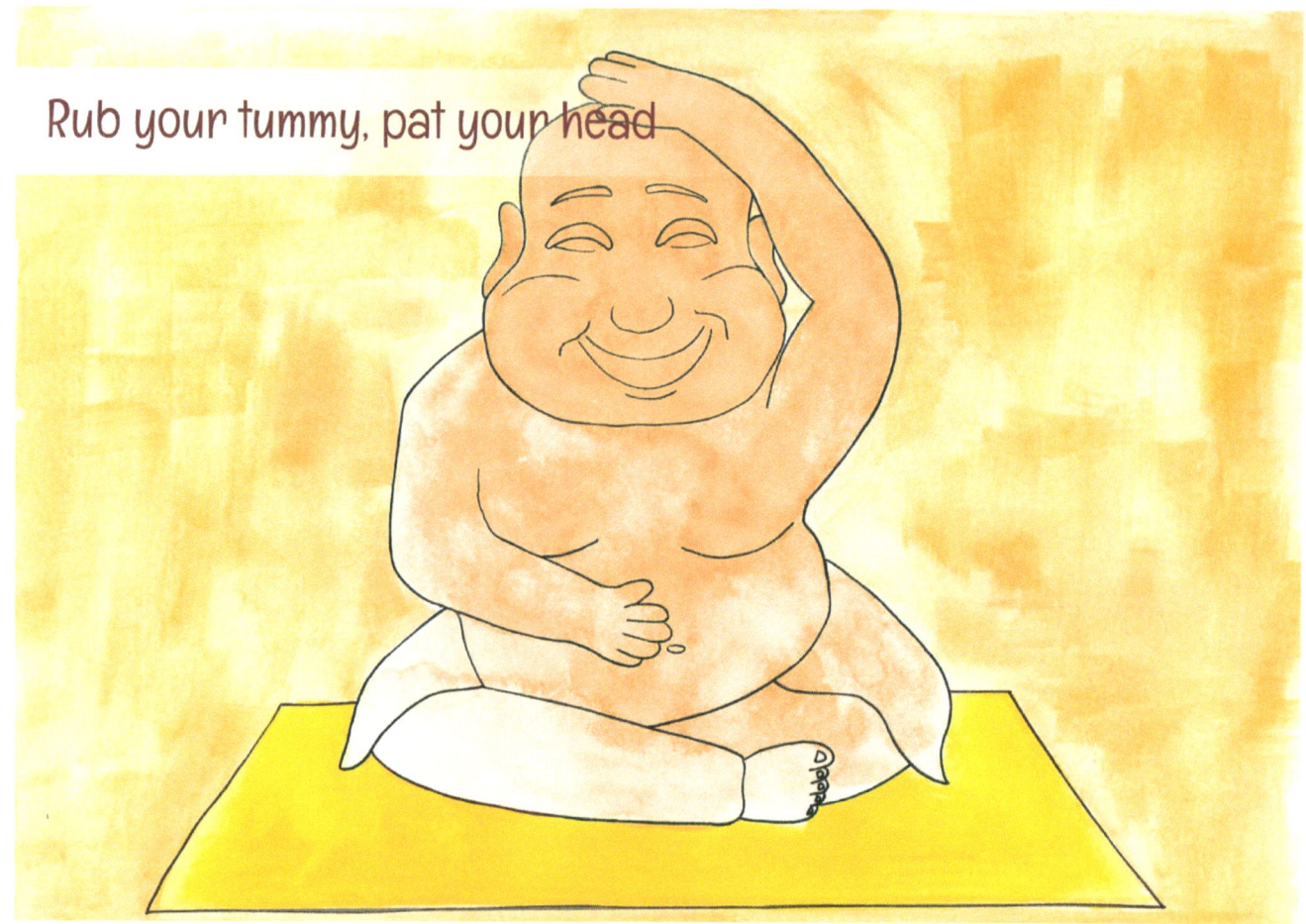

Both of your brain hemispheres are involved in most mental processes you engage in, and information is constantly being sent back and forth between them. The cooperation between the right and left brain is essential for us to learn better, function more intelligently, and become proficient in anything. Whatever it is you are engaged in — reading, writing, music, art, sports — each hemisphere has something important to contribute for you to have access to both technique and inspiration. Mismatching the movements of your hands and/or feet is a good brain exercise that promotes coordination and cooperation between the two brain hemispheres.

HOW TO: Place your right hand on your belly and your left hand on your head. Breathe comfortably and start rubbing your belly while patting your head. Do it for two to three minutes, and then switch sides.

Additional content: Right-left brain integration yoga practice (video) + blog post

NOTES

"In order to live balanced, meaningful, and creative lives full of connected relationships, it's crucial that our two hemispheres work together."
— David Siegel and Tina Payne Bryson, *The Whole Brain Child*

Tend the garden of your mind

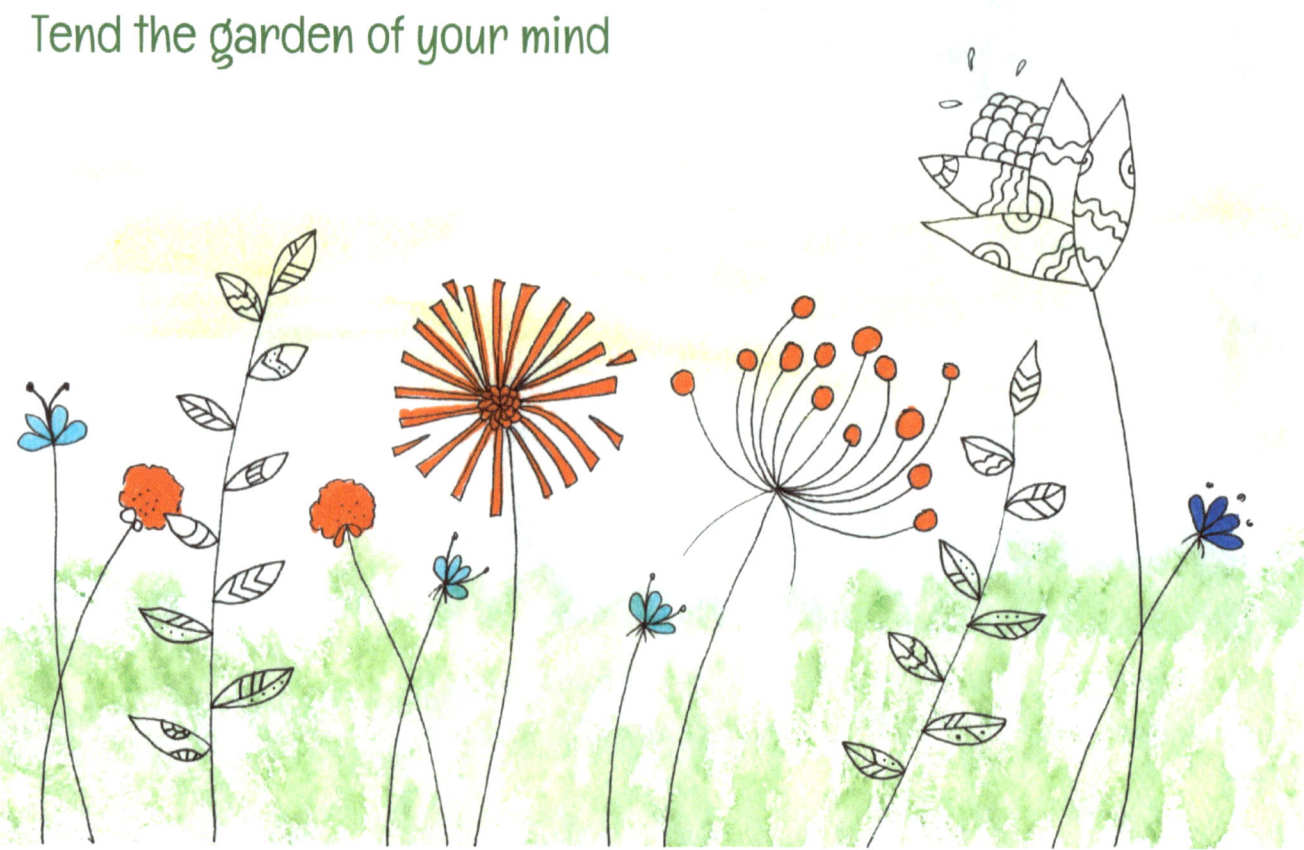

We all fall into a trap of running negative stories in our minds. Once we hook into those patterns of thought, they begin to run on a loop, and it becomes too difficult to get out. Jill Bolte Taylor in her book *My Stroke of Insight* writes: "The more aware I remain about what my brain is saying and how those thoughts feel inside my body, the more I own my power in choosing what I want to spend my time thinking about and how I want to feel. If I want to retain my inner peace, I must be willing to consistently and persistently TEND THE GARDEN OF MY MIND moment by moment, and be willing to make the decision a thousand times a day." To break out of the pattern of negative self-talk, she recommends switching your thinking to one of three things:

- Remember something that you find fascinating and ponder it more deeply.
- Think about something that gives you great joy.
- Think about something that you would like to do.

Try those strategies to break the patterns of your negative thinking.

HOW TO

Next time when you notice yourself getting stuck in a mental loop of negative self-talk, instead of getting caught up in it, try to think of something that you find interesting, or something that gives you joy, or simply direct your attention toward something you want to do. Experiment with those options and see which one seems the most effective for you.

NOTES

"Step one to experiencing inner peace is the willingness to be present in the right here, right now."
— Jill Bolte Taylor, *My Stroke of Insight*

Chant for mental clarity

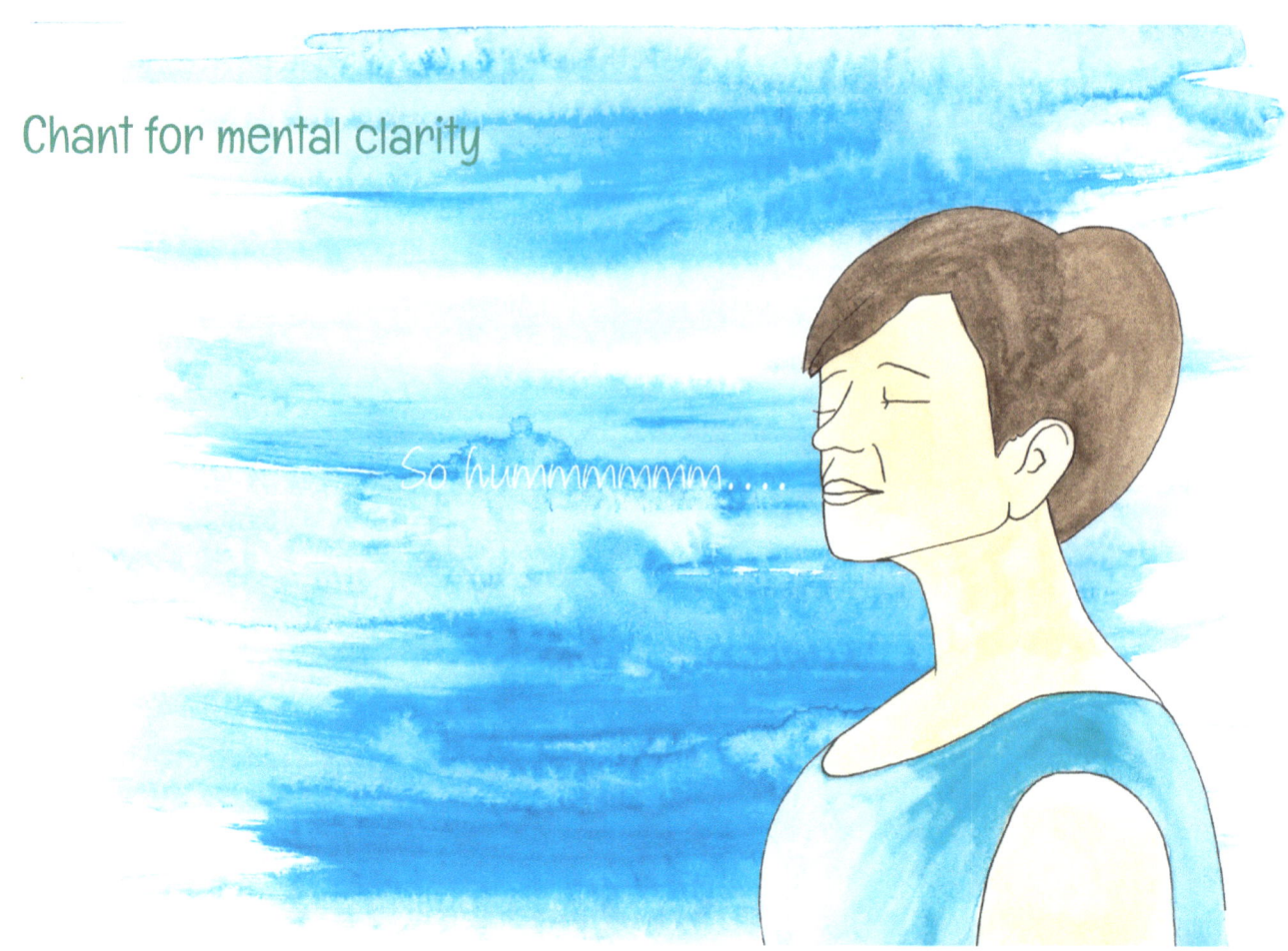

So hummmmmm....

You know how sometimes you get a song stuck in your head? You just keep singing it in a loop, overriding other loops in your brain. But instead of a silly song, you can choose a chant that actually means something to you and that can uplift you. It can be anything you like — a line from a poem, a phrase, a quote, or a mantra. My yoga teacher Gary Kraftsow says that chanting can be used as a "digestive enzyme to metabolize our neurosis." Through speech we process things, and using a mantra speeds up the process.

HOW TO: Pick a line from a poem, a phrase, a quote, or a mantra. Mentally say part of it as you inhale and part of it as you exhale. (For a short quote, repeat the whole thing on inhale and the whole thing on exhale.) For example, IN (say mentally): "This, too, shall pass." EX: (say mentally): "This, too, shall pass." Repeat it for at least 12 breaths and see if the negative pattern that runs through your mind is replaced by something positive.

Additional content: Hrdavam Mavi chant (video)

NOTES

Make "My Happy Place" playlist

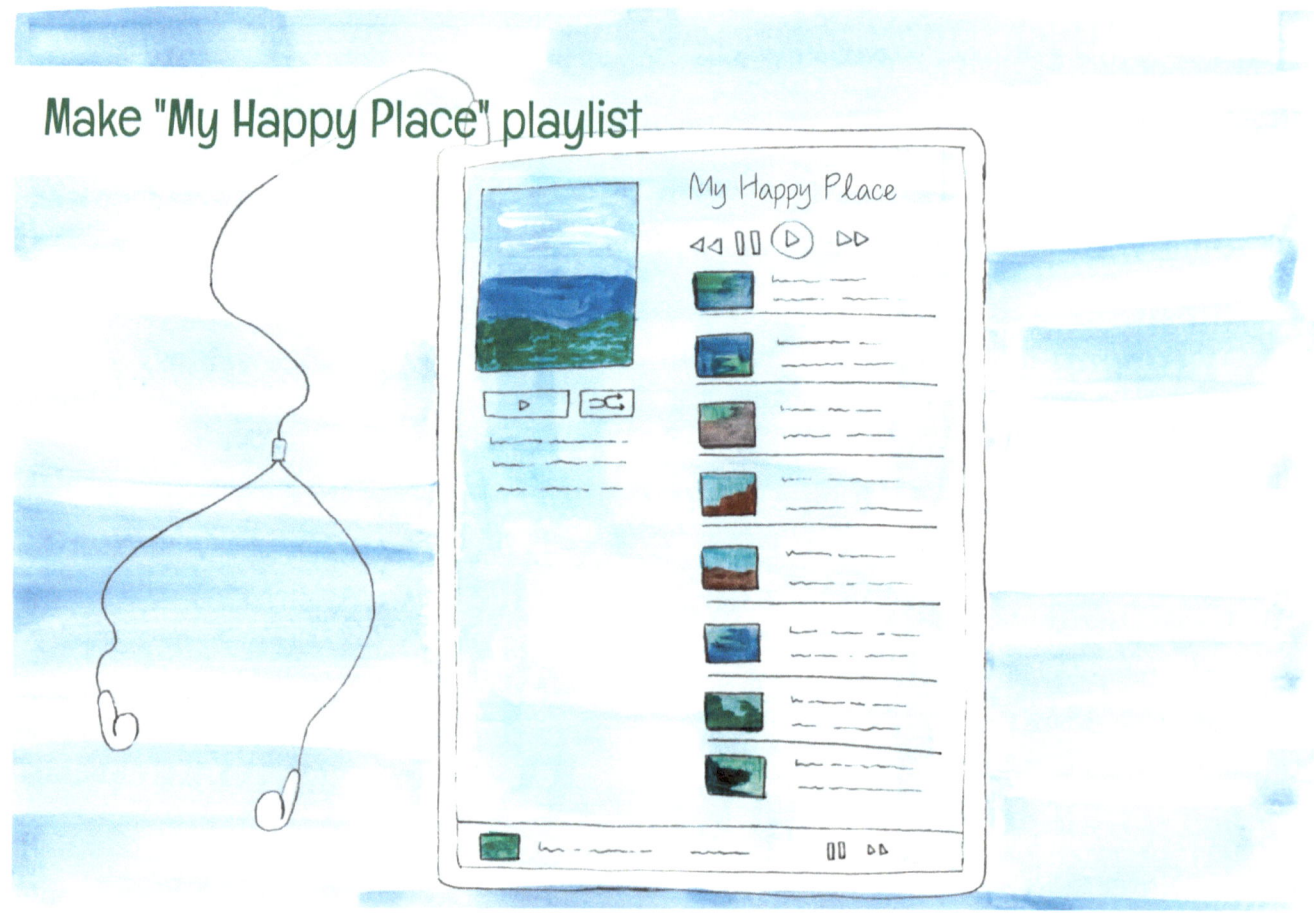

You don't need to be a scientist to know that sound (music and singing) has a profound effect on the way we feel, often in a predictable way. For example, you probably won't fall asleep when you listen to a marching band, nor would you jump around wildly when you listen to a lullaby. French otolaryngologist Alfred A. Tomatis has suggested that the primary function of the ear is to provide the cells of the body with electrical stimulation or cortical charge. He differentiates between "charging sounds" that promote more dynamism and energy and "dis-charging sounds" that rid you of access energy and have a more calming effect.

HOW TO: Create a soundtrack for your day. How do you want to feel? Choose songs from your collection or any online streaming service to create a playlist of songs that give you the feeling you are looking for. Play it during the day and see if it has an impact on how you feel.

🖱 Additional content: sample "My Happy Place" playlist (Spotify) + blog post about effects of sound

NOTES

Rediscover your creativity

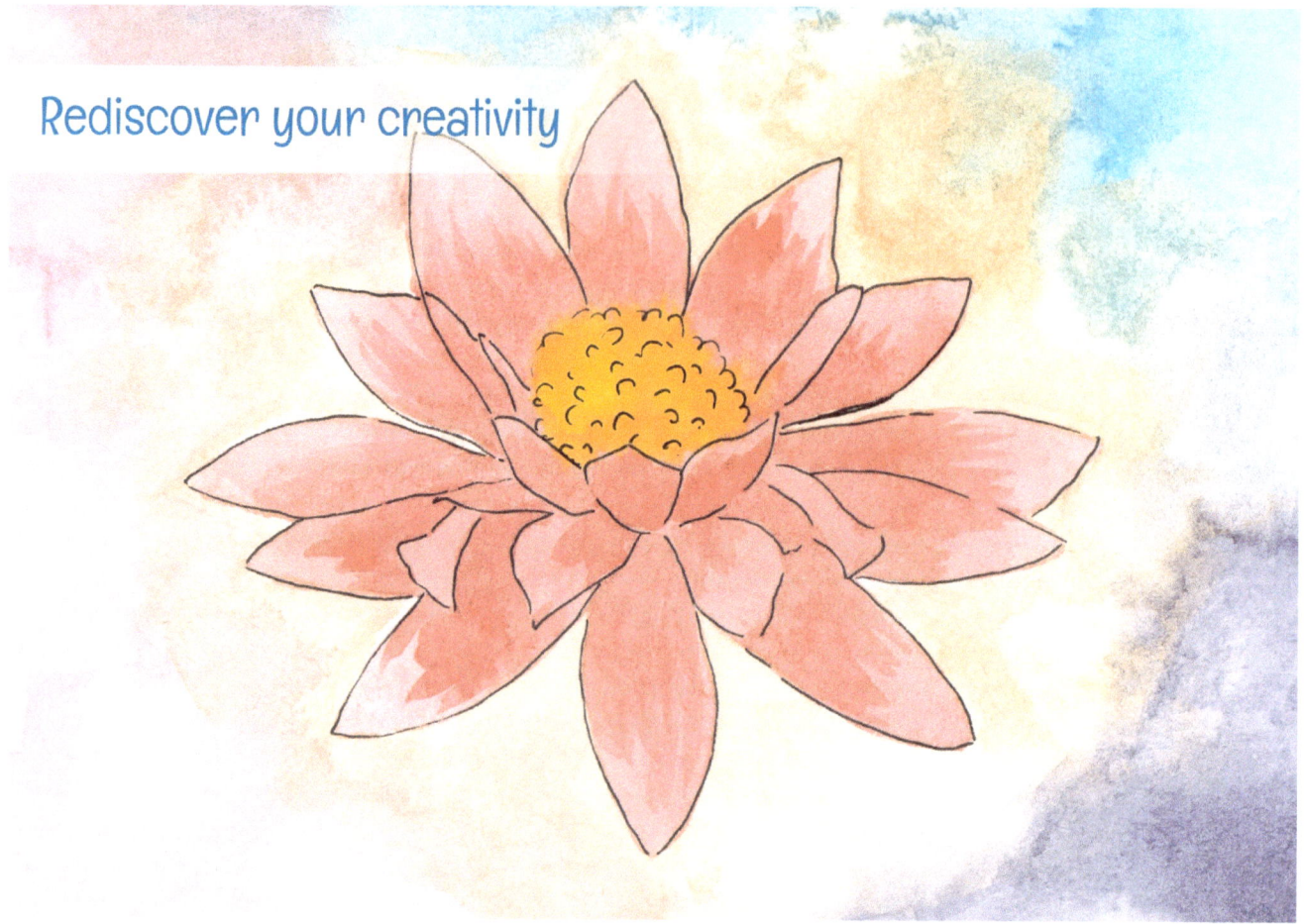

When was the last time you did something creative just because it gave you joy? Do you view creativity as an indulgence or a necessary part of your life? Time and time again, I hear some version of this from my students: "I used to love painting, climbing, making jewelry, going to theater, writing, etc., but I just don't have time to do this anymore." Let's make some space for something creative that gives you joy.

HOW TO: Reflect for a moment: what are some of the things you used to do just for fun that you do not do anymore? Think of one activity that used to give you joy and make a plan for when you will do it this week. Set aside some time and when the time comes — dive in!

NOTES

"An abiding stereotype of creativity is that it turns people crazy.
I disagree: Not expressing creativity turns people crazy."
— Elizabeth Gilbert, *Big Magic: Creative Living Beyond Fear*

Set a date with yourself

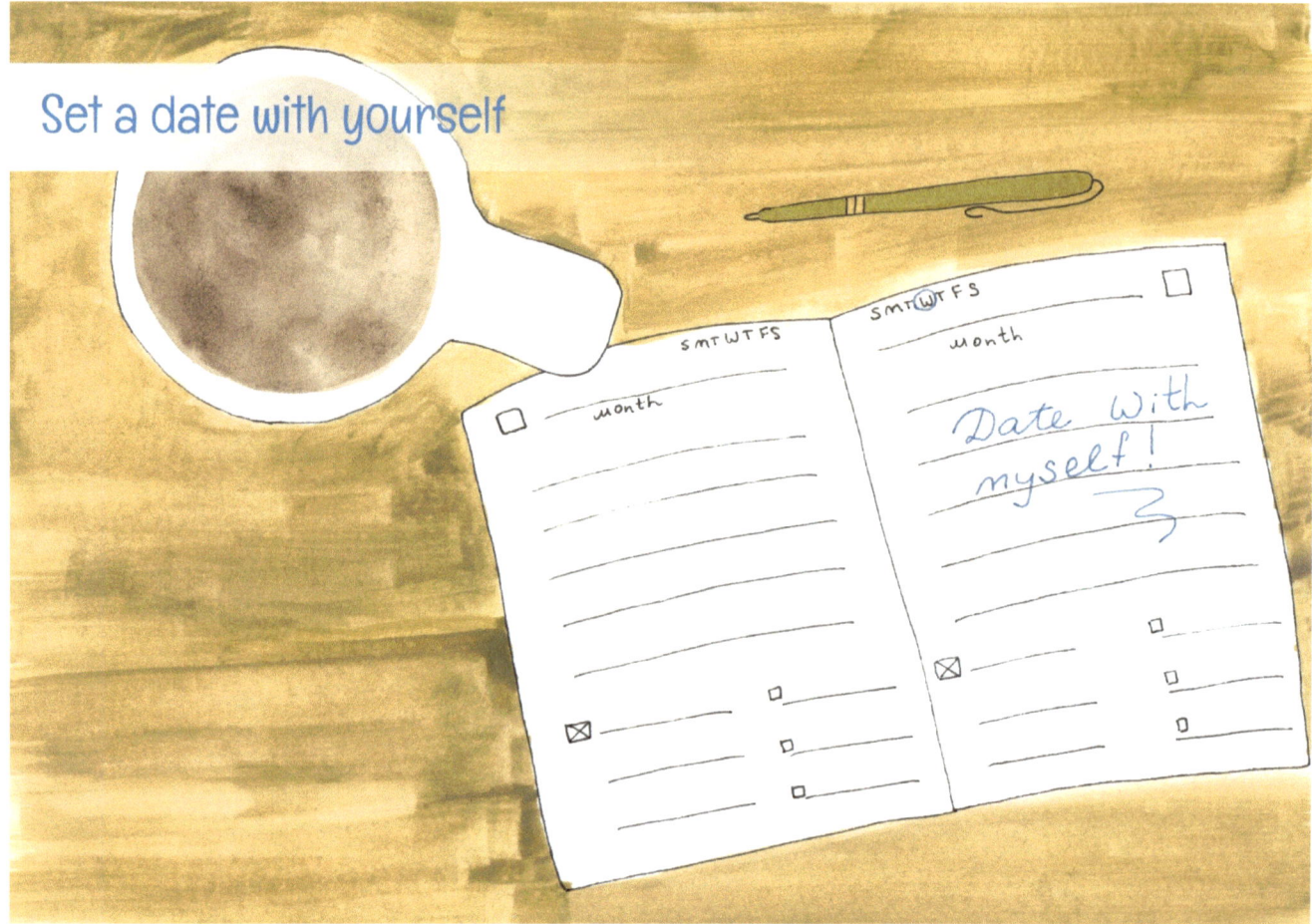

Sometimes, we wear our "busyness" as a badge of honor, but constantly moving from one thing to the next can rob us of our ability to play, create, or simply think. Set aside some time to slow down and have a date with yourself.

HOW TO: Look at your calendar and schedule an hour sometime during the week for a date with yourself. Please take it seriously. When the time comes, start the hour by sitting quietly, closing your eyes, and asking yourself "What kind of activity would nourish my soul?" It can be a creative pursuit or some quiet time to just sit and think about where you are and where you are going; you can have tea, write in your journal, or read an interesting book, taking time to reflect on what you are reading. Whatever it is that you are drawn to and that makes you feel warm and fuzzy inside, do it for the next hour without guilt. Afterwards, notice how it affects your state of mind for the rest of the day.

NOTES

"By all means, do not let me or anyone else ever take away your suffering if you are committed to it!"
— Elizabeth Gilbert *Big Magic: Creative Living Beyond Fear*

Envision the big picture

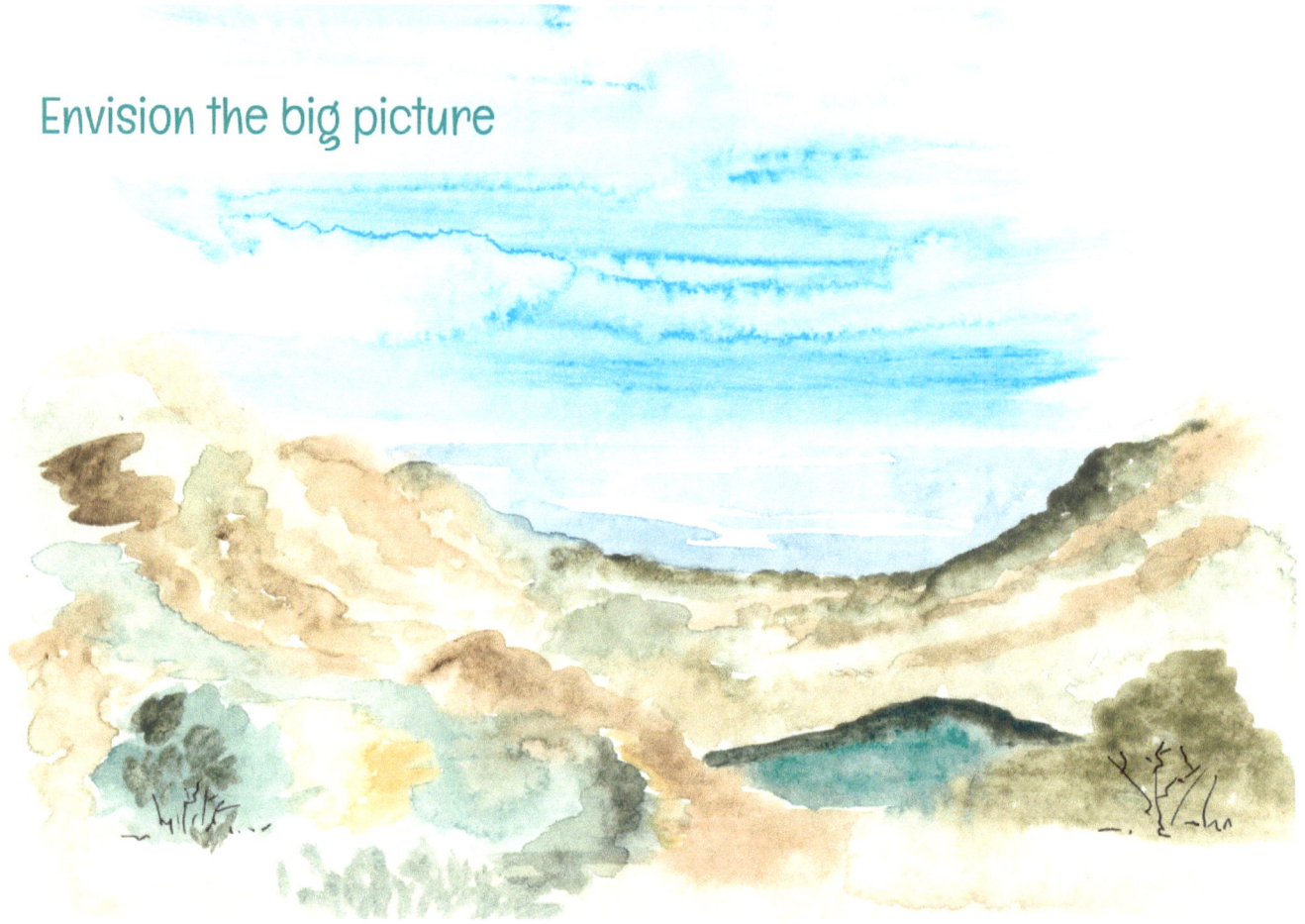

The ultimate purpose of yoga is to facilitate mental clarity. One of the ways to do that is to encourage ourselves to reassess how we engage with our life in the moment. You can use meditation to step back, loosen the grip a bit, and envision what kind of feeling you want your life to give you. Try this guided meditation to identify the relationships and activities that already give you that feeling to emphasize them in your life.

HOW TO: Get settled in a comfortable seated position. Close your eyes and begin to deepen your inhalation and lengthen your exhalation. As you continue to breathe comfortably, bring your attention to the quality of your mental activity. How does it feel to you right now? Then bring your attention to your chest. How does it feel? How does breathing feel? Drop your attention down to your belly. How does your belly feel? Does it move with your breath? How does your body feel overall? Is there tension or restraint of any sort? Breathe with that awareness.

NOTES

What kind of physical discomfort do you experience day after day?

What do you think is the reason for it?

What kind of activities makes it feel worse? How often do you do them?

What kind of activities makes it feel better? How often do you do them?

What kind of actions have you taken to deal with the issue?

What kind of professionals have you seen so far to help you deal with that issue (doctor, PT, LMT, etc.)?

What is the next step you need to take to address this issue?

When will you take that step?

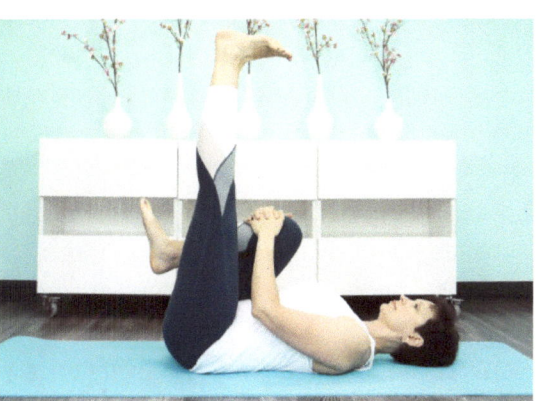

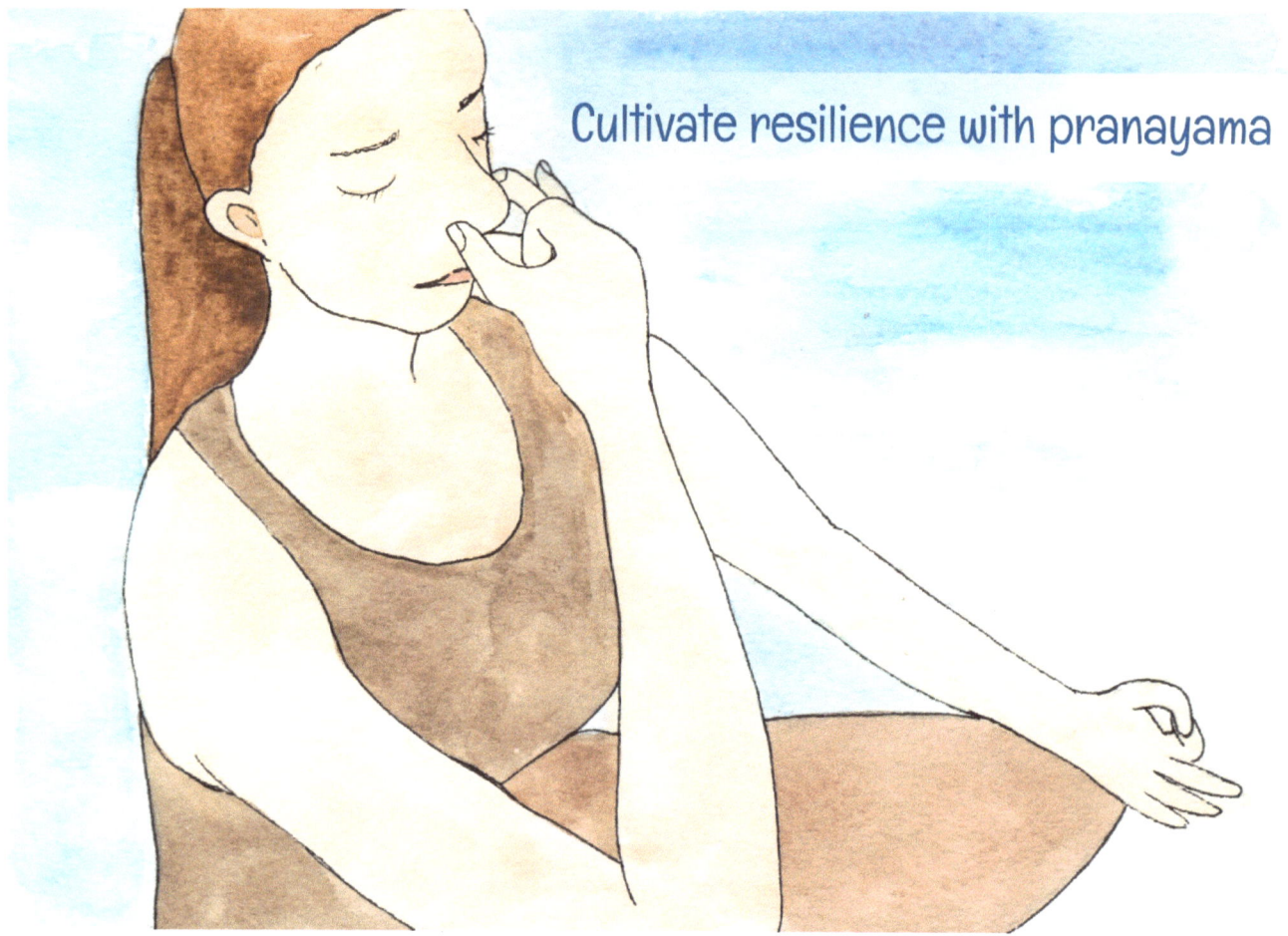

Cultivate resilience with pranayama

According to the viniyoga tradition, our aging process is represented by the movement of sun throughout the day. Sunrise represents childhood, midday represents adult life, and sunset represents old age. Most of us fall into the mid-day stage of life (the "householder" stage, roughly 25 to 70 years old). At this stage, we need more focus on energy management practices to support us in our busy lives, which likely include careers, children, aging parents, and households. During this time, our yoga practice needs to help us cultivate physical, physiological, mental, and emotional resilience. It cannot drain our energy but needs to support and enhance it. Pranayama by definition means "life force expansion." For "householders," regular pranayama is the most important part of the yoga practice.

HOW TO: Include pranayama in every yoga practice you do. It can range from deep conscious breathing to specific pranayama techniques. Take at least 12 breaths with your chosen technique.

🖱 Additional content: suggestions for yoga practices that revolve around pranayama

NOTES

Out with the old, in with the new

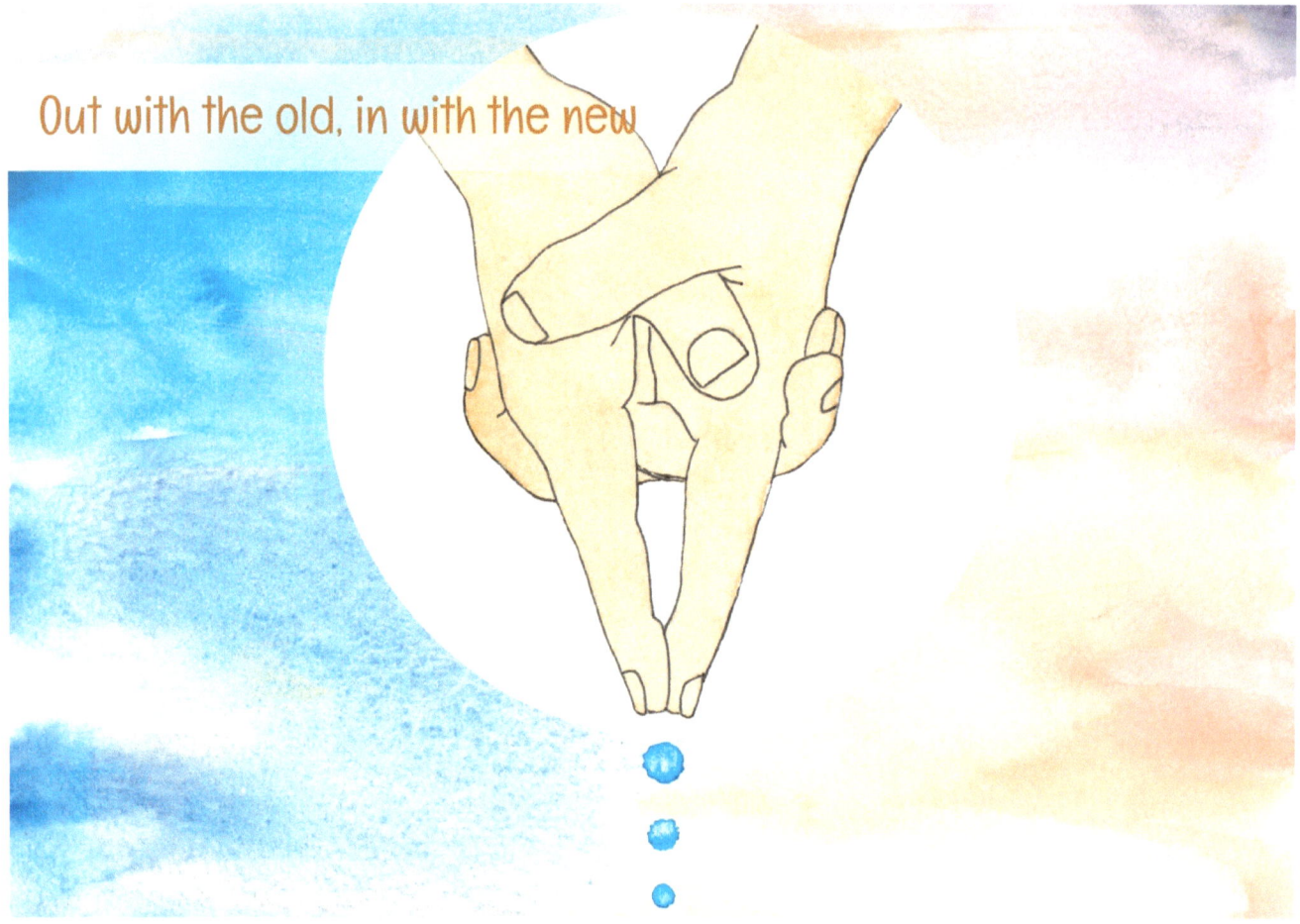

Disproportionally large areas of our brains are dedicated to processing motor and sensory signals from our hands, which make our hands powerful communication tools. Hand gestures can be used to evoke specific meaning, and in yoga, those gestures are called "mudras." Each mudra represents a "core quality." Joseph and Lilian Le Page write: "These qualities are reflections of our deeper spiritual essence, which is already present as a potential, ready to be awakened. Mudras function as energetic keys that unlock those qualities."

HOW TO: Ksepana Mudra represents the quality of letting go. Interlace the fingers of both hands and extend both index fingers. Cross the thumbs on top of each other. Rest your hands on your lap pointing the index fingers down. Close your eyes and focus on your breath. Every time you inhale, imagine gathering old stale energy within your body, and on the exhale, imagine pouring it out of your system through the arms, hands, and fingers. Take 12 breaths like that. Then place your hands on your knees, palms up, and with every inhalation, imagine receiving new fresh energy through your hands.

NOTES

Journal about your yoga practice

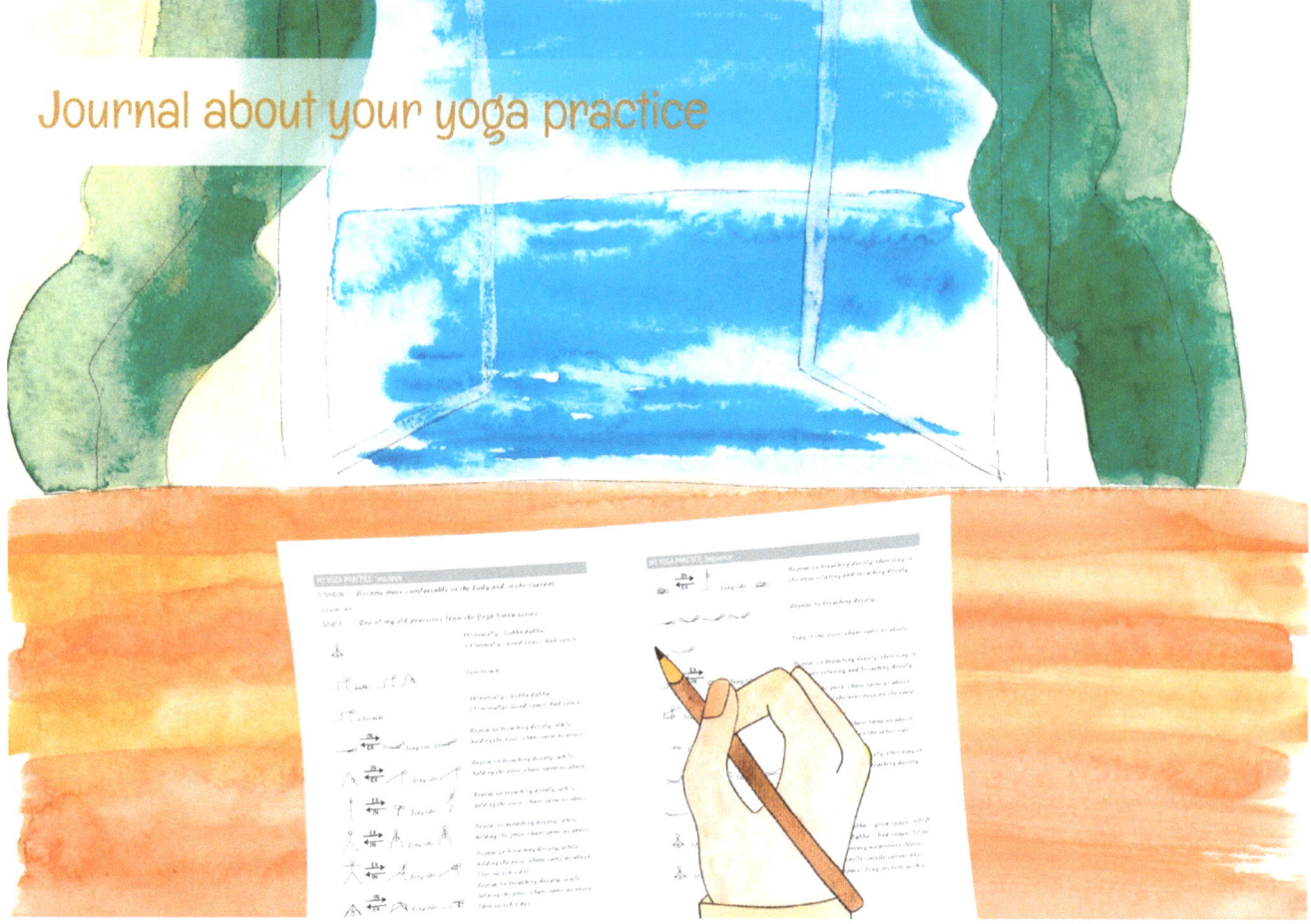

If you ever kept a journal, you know that putting your feelings into words and writing them down help you better understand what's going on. It also helps to diminish the negative charge associated with life challenges. In a similar way, keeping records of your yoga practice in written form helps you process your response to the practice and to document your progress. It is particularly useful if you are trying to investigate a specific set of practices, test certain techniques, or consistently work on a chronic problem.

HOW TO: After you finish your yoga practice, take few moments to write down the main idea of the practice and whether or not it met your current needs. What seemed most effective? What didn't work at all? What changes are needed to make it more effective?

🖱 Additional content: sample pages from Personal Yoga Practice Journal

NOTES

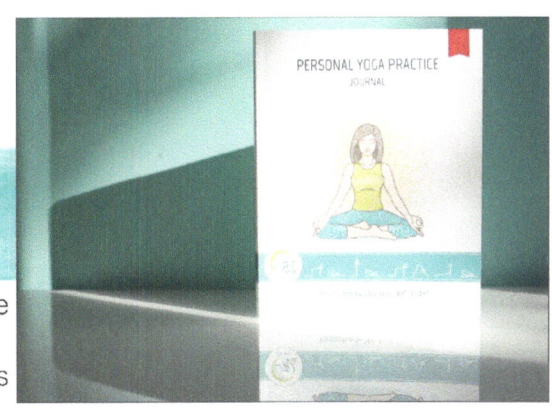

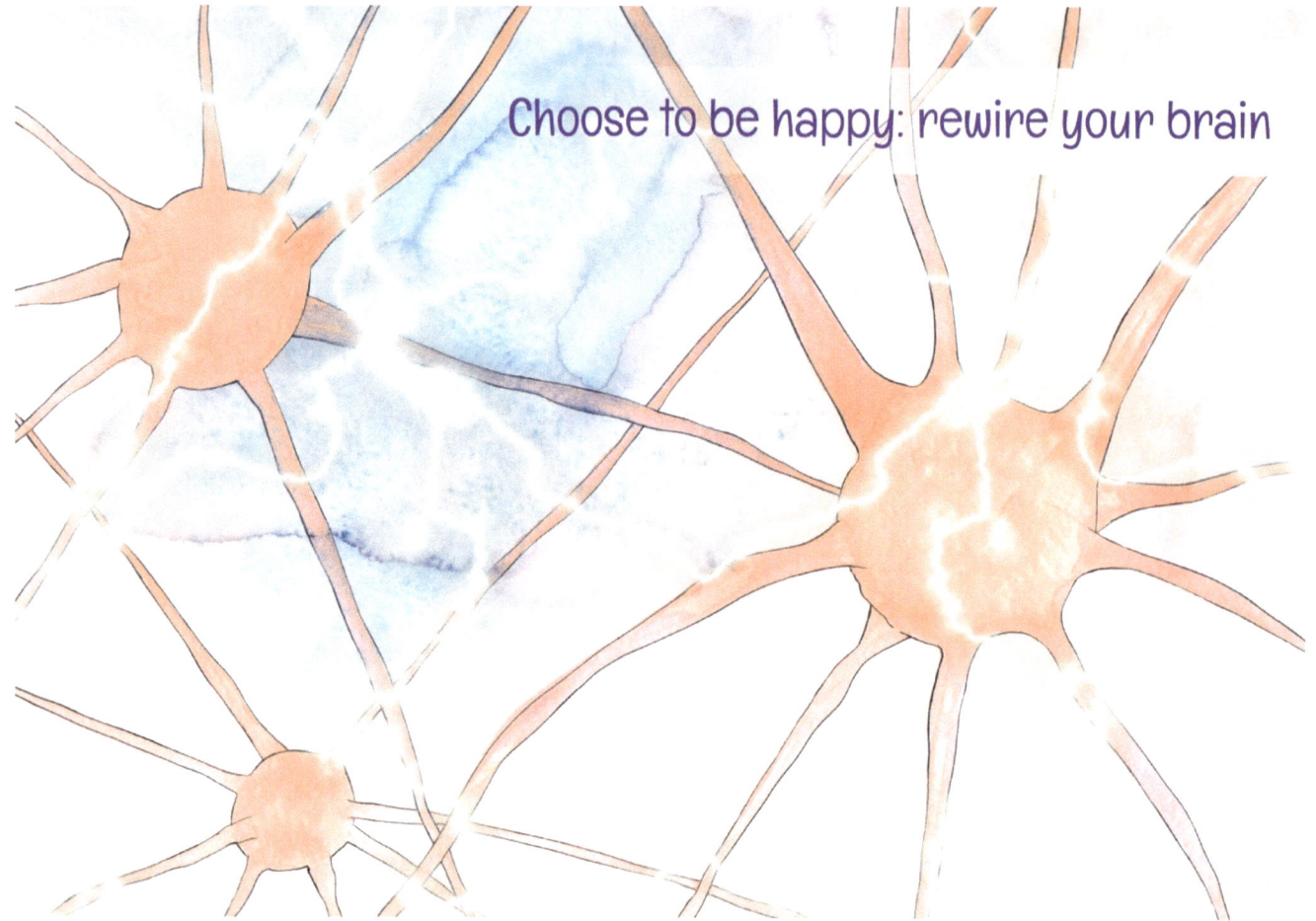

Choose to be happy: rewire your brain

The wiring of your brain is constantly changing in response to how you use it. In *Hardwiring Happiness*, Rick Hanson writes: "If you keep resting your mind on self-criticism, worries, grumbling about others, hurts, and stress, then your brain will be shaped into greater reactivity, vulnerability to anxiety and depressed mood, a narrow focus on threats and losses, and inclinations toward anger, sadness, and guilt. On the other hand, if you keep resting your mind on good events and conditions (someone was nice to you, there's a roof over your head), pleasant feelings, the things you do get done, physical pleasures, and your good intentions and qualities, then over time your brain will take a different shape, one with strength and resilience hardwired into it, as well as a realistically optimistic outlook, a positive mood, and a sense of worth." The choice is yours.

HOW TO: Every time you have a positive experience, make a conscious effort to *install* it in your brain. To do that, first focus on fully experiencing it through your senses, linger with it for 5 to 10 seconds to savor it, and then imagine yourself absorbing it into your body and your brain.

NOTES

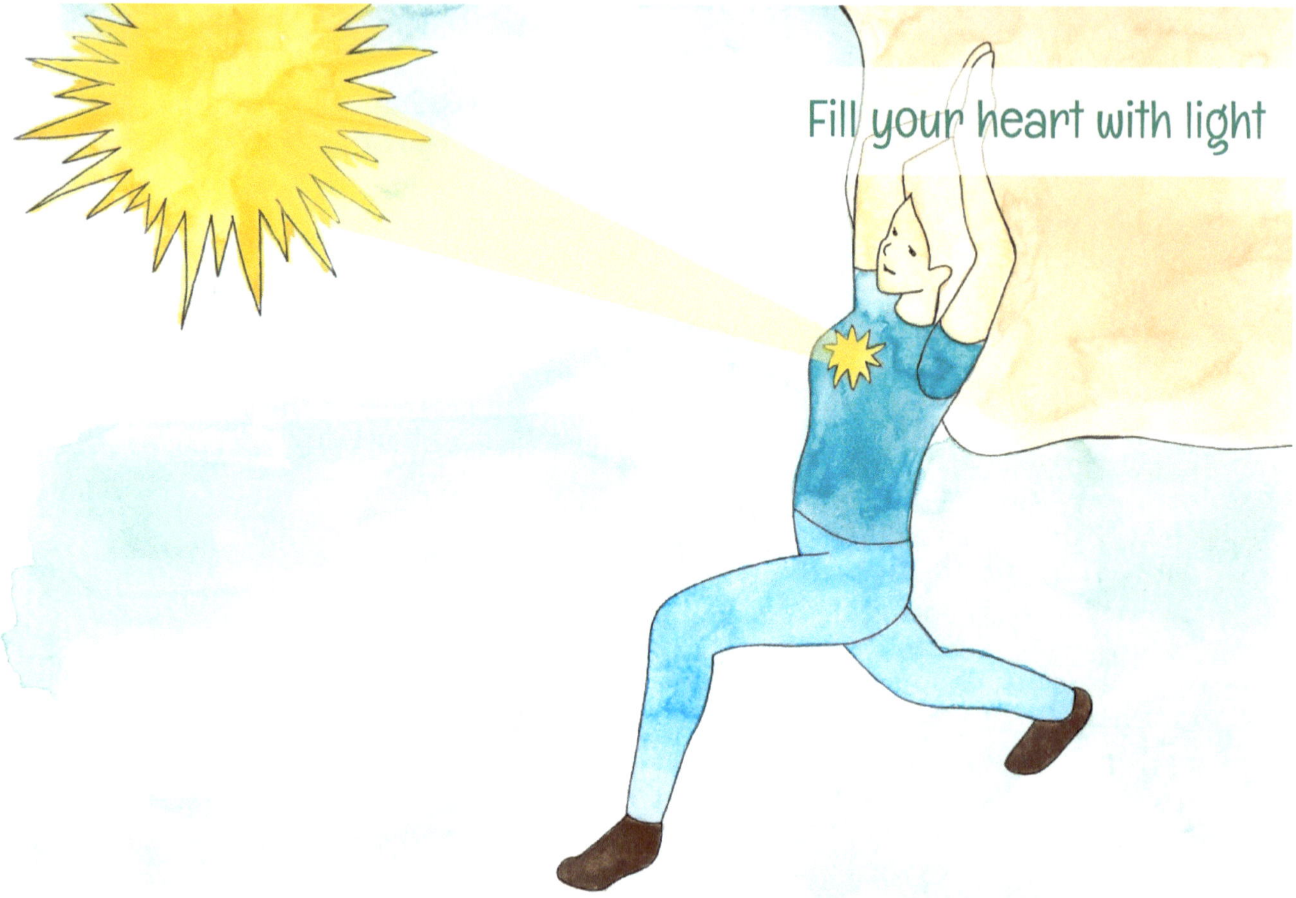

Fill your heart with light

1   Get settled in a comfortable seated position, deepen your breath. As you continue to breathe, take a moment to notice how the area around your heart feels right now. Does it feel spacious and courageous or guarded and timid? Take few breaths with that awareness.

2   **EX**   **IN**   CAT-COW. Begin on your hands and knees. IN: Lift the chest and chin. EX: Round the back and tuck the chin in. Focus on expanding your ribcage (front and back) as you move. Repeat 4x.

3   **IN**   **EX**   **IN**   **EX**   VAJRASANA. Begin on your knees with the chest over the thighs and hands on the lower back. IN: Lift up, bringing your arms up. EX: Place the hands on the opposite shoulders, round the upper back a bit, and tuck the chin in. IN: Bring the arms out, widening the chest. EX: Move back down, placing hands on your back. Repeat 3x.

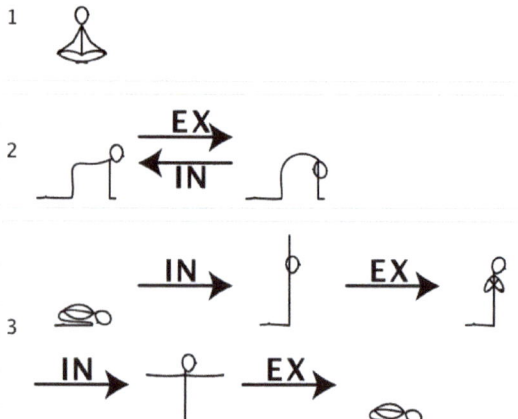

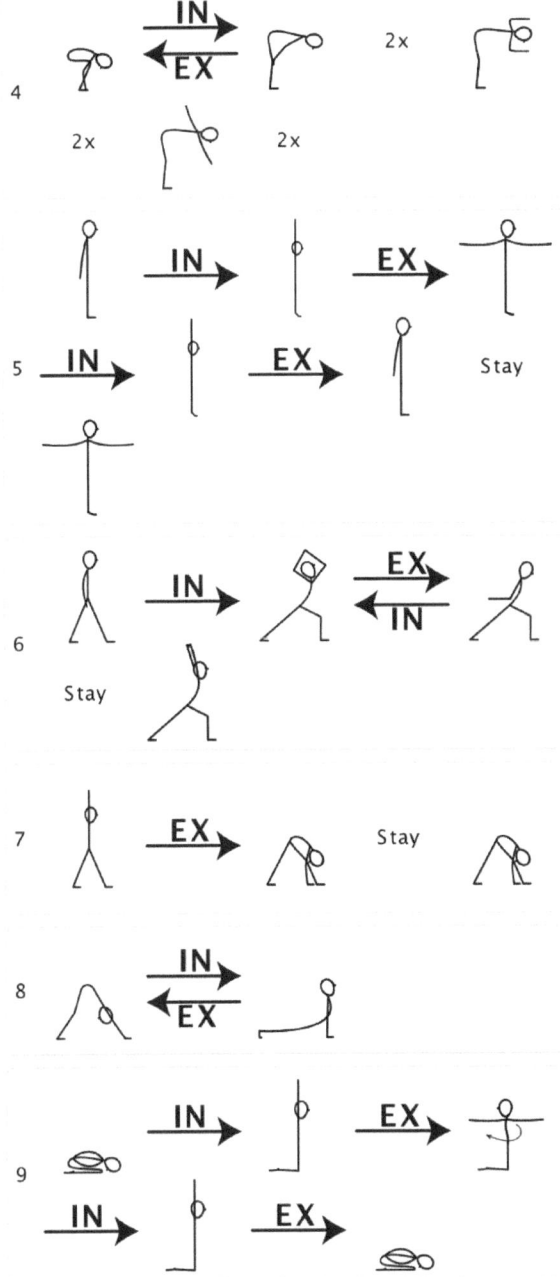

ARDHA UTTANASANA. Begin with your knees bent, chest over your thighs. IN: Extend the legs and flatten your back, keeping your hands on your shins EX: Bend down, moving the chest toward the thighs. Repeat 2x. Next time lift the upper body about halfway up, bending the elbows out to the sides. Repeat 2x. Next time, lift the upper body about halfway up, extending your arms out to the sides. Repeat 2x. Transition into standing.

TADASANA HEEL RAISES. Begin standing with your feet hip distance apart. IN: Sweep the arms up lifting up on the balls of the feet. EX: Lower the heels slightly down, arms out to the sides. IN: Lift back up, arms up. EX: Bring your heels and arms down. Repeat 3x, then stay on your toes with arms extended out for 3 deep breaths.

VIRABHADRASANA 1. Begin standing with feet hip distance apart, one foot forward, arms down. IN: Bend the front knee as you move the arms up into a diamond shape, look up. EX: Keep the front knee bent, move your elbows toward the waist, and look down. Repeat 3x, then extend the arms up and take 3 full deep breaths. Do # 7, then switch sides.

PARSVOTTANASANA. Begin standing with your right foot forward and both arms up. EX: Contract your abdomen and bend forward, keeping your spine long. Place your hands on the ground and drape your chest over your thigh (bend the front knee if necessary. IN: Expand your upper back. EX: Relax your neck and shoulders. 4 breaths.

ARDHA MUKHA SVANASANA/URDVA MUKHA SVANASANA. Begin on your hands and feet. IN: Carry your upper body forward to align the shoulders over the hips, and lower your hips down while lifting the chest forward. EX: Push your hips back, stretching from the hands to the tailbone. Repeat 3x

VAJRASANA. Begin on your knees with the chest over the thighs and hands on the lower back. IN: Lift up, sweeping the arms up. EX: Turn to your right, arms out to the sides, look back. IN: Return to the center, arms up. EX: Turn to your left, arms out to the sides, look back. IN: Return to the center, arms up. Move back down, placing your hands on your back. Be sure to pull the belly in when you twist. Repeat 3x.

The practice continues on the next page >

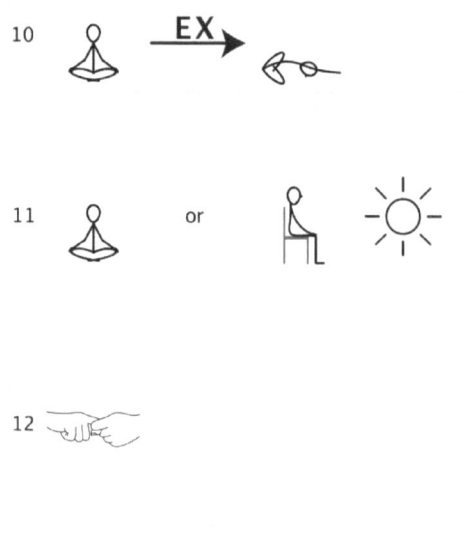

10 SUKHASANA. Sit with your legs crossed. EX: Walk your hands forward and bend down. Support yourself with your hands, relax your neck, and breathe into your upper back. 4 breaths.

11 or PRANAYAMA. Get settled in a comfortable seated position of your choice. Deepen your breath. IN: Expand your ribcage in every direction. EX: Relax your shoulders. 6 breaths.
Sense the position of the sun right now. If you can see the light, become aware of it with your eyes closed. If you cannot see the light, imagine it. IN: Imagine breathing in the light and filling up your ribcage. Pause for a moment. EX: Imagine the light seeping from your ribcage into the rest of your body. Continue to breathe like that for 6 breaths.

12 TARJANI MUDRA instills a sense of awareness and openness on the chest, heart, and lungs. | Hold your hands in front of the solar plexus with elbows slightly out. Curl the fingers of both hands in and interlace the index fingers, while pulling them slightly apart. Take 6 deep breaths here cultivating the sensation of spaciousness around your heart.

FINAL CHECK IN. Rest your hands on your knees and take a few more deep breaths. Notice how you feel.

13

Additional content: Fill your heart with light practice (video)

NOTES

NOTES

References

1. *The Year of Pleasures: A Novel* by Elizabeth Berg, Random House, 2005
2. *Eat, Pray, Love: One Woman's Search for Everything Across Italy, India and Indonesia* by Elizabeth Gilbert, Riverhead Books, 2006
3. *Happy Yoga: 7 Reasons There is Nothing to Worry About* by Steve Ross, HarperCollins Publishers, 2003
4. *Presence: Bringing Your Boldest Self to Your Biggest Challenges* by Amy Cuddy, Little, Brown and Company, 2015
5. *The Happiness Advantage: How a positive Brain Fuels Success in Work and Life* by Shawn Achor, Currency, 2010
6. *My Stroke of Insight: A Brain Scientist's Personal Journey* by Jill Bolte Taylor, Viking, 2006
7. *The Whole Brain Child: 12 Revolutionary Strategies to Nurture Your Child's Developing Mind* by David Siegel and Tina Payne Bryson, Delacorte Press, 2011
8. *Big Magic: Creative Living Beyond Fear* by Elizabeth Gilbert, Riverhead Books, 2015
9. *Mudras for Healing and Transformation* by Joseph and Lilian Le Page, Integrative Yoga Therapy, 2014
10. *Hardwiring Happiness: The New Brain Science of Contentment, Calm, and Confidence* by Rick Hanson, Harmony, 2013